Inherited Blood Disorders - Advances in Diagnosis and Treatment

Edited by Silva Zupančić Šalek

Published in London, United Kingdom

Inherited Blood Disorders - Advances in Diagnosis and Treatment
http://dx.doi.org/10.5772/intechopen.1004471
Edited by Silva Zupančić Šalek

Contributors
Ali A. Alyahawi, Amar Narayan Shrestha, Behzad Davarnia, Giancarlo Castaman, Gulsum Feyza Turkes, Jolana Schmiedl, Mahdi Karimi, Mohammed Abdulwahid Almorish, Mohammed AW. Almorish, Sara Arish, Sindhu Gyawali, Zeynep Ece Demirbaş

First published in London, United Kingdom, 2025 by IntechOpen
IntechOpen is the global imprint of INTECHOPEN LIMITED, registered in England and Wales, registration number: 11086078, 167-169 Great Portland Street, London, W1W 5PF, United Kingdom

For EU product safety concerns: IN TECH d.o.o., Prolaz Marije Krucifikse Kozulić 3, 51000 Rijeka, Croatia, info@intechopen.com or visit our website at intechopen.com.

British Library Cataloguing-in-Publication Data
A catalogue record for this book is available from the British Library

Inherited Blood Disorders - Advances in Diagnosis and Treatment
Edited by Silva Zupančić Šalek
p. cm.
Print ISBN 978-1-83634-275-5
Online ISBN 978-1-83634-274-8
eBook (PDF) ISBN 978-1-83634-276-2

Meet the editor

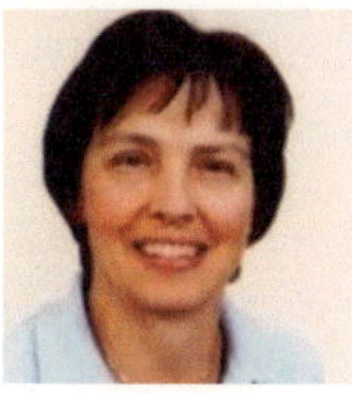

Professor Silva Zupančić Šalek obtained her Medical Degree at the School of Medicine, University of Zagreb, followed by an MSc in 1986 and a Ph.D. in 2004. She completed her specialization in Internal Medicine and Hematology. Her professional career was primarily based at the University Hospital Centre Zagreb, where she served as Head of the Division for Haemostasis, Thrombosis and Benign Hematopoietic Disorders, as well as Head of the Reference Centre for Haemophilia and Haemostatic Disorders. From 2016 to 2017, she served as Head of the Division of Hematology in the Department of Internal Medicine. She is currently a Full Professor of Internal Medicine at the University of Josip Juraj Strossmayer in Osijek and the University of Zagreb School of Medicine. Since 2020, she has been working as a Scientific Adviser and Consultant Hematologist at the Clinical Hospital Sveti Duh, Zagreb. Her scientific and clinical work has focused on hereditary and acquired haemostatic disorders, platelet diseases, thrombosis and hemoglobinopathies. She established the National Haemophilia Centre, organized the Registry of Patients with Bleeding Disorders, and significantly improved the treatment of haemophilia through the introduction of novel therapies. She received the World Federation of Haemophilia Award for outstanding contributions in the diagnosis and treatment of haemophilia and completed a WFH fellowship at the Oxford Haemophilia and Thrombosis Centre. Prof. Silva Zupančić Šalek has led over 22 clinical trials as principal investigator and published more than 180 peer-reviewed articles.

Contents

Preface

Inherited blood disorders represent a heterogeneous group of genetic conditions that primarily affect red blood cells, hemoglobin synthesis, coagulation factors, and erythrocyte enzymatic pathways. This volume places particular emphasis on hemoglobinopathies, with a detailed focus on sickle cell disease and thalassemia, while also addressing broader hematological topics such as postpartum hemorrhage and neutropenia.

At the outset, particular attention is given to the molecular structure of hemoglobin and the therapeutic innovations that have arisen from this knowledge. Mutations in globin genes lead to structural and functional abnormalities of hemoglobin, resulting in disorders such as sickle cell disease and thalassemia. A deep understanding of the genetic and molecular mechanisms involved, including alterations in transcription, RNA splicing, and protein stability, has been crucial for the development of targeted therapies. Current approaches range from traditional interventions, such as blood transfusions and iron chelation therapy, to advanced molecular strategies including genome editing with CRISPR/Cas9. These innovations open the door to the possibility of correcting the underlying genetic defect and achieving a functional cure.

Diagnostic advancements have also been remarkable. While traditional methods, such as hemoglobin electrophoresis, high-performance liquid chromatography, and isoelectric focusing, remain the gold standard, new technologies are increasingly complementing and enhancing clinical practice. Point-of-care diagnostic devices now allow for rapid and affordable detection of hemoglobin variants, particularly in low-resource settings, thereby expanding access to early diagnosis. In parallel, genetic testing and next-generation sequencing enable the precise identification of mutations, facilitating prenatal and carrier screening, as well as improving the early recognition of disease. Such progress not only increases diagnostic accuracy but also facilitates earlier intervention and better outcomes for patients.

In the treatment of sickle cell disease, significant progress has been achieved through both pharmacological agents and gene therapy. Novel drugs reduce the frequency of vaso-occlusive crises and disease-related complications, while hematopoietic stem cell transplantation remains the only established curative option, though limited by donor availability and procedural risks. Emerging gene therapies—both gene addition and gene-editing approaches—are redefining the therapeutic landscape and offering hope for long-term correction of the disease. Comparable advances have also been made in β-thalassemia major, where modern molecular testing is now integrated with improved strategies for monitoring and managing iron overload.

Nutritional therapy is another key aspect addressed in this book, underscoring the importance of individualized dietary interventions for patients with hemoglobinopathies. Adjustments in macronutrient intake, combined with essential micronutrients such as iron, folic acid, and vitamin D, play a crucial role in comprehensive care. Looking ahead, nutritional support is expected to become an integral part of standard clinical practice, implemented through a multidisciplinary approach.

Technological innovations, including the development of automated haematology analysers and digital peripheral smear devices, have further enhanced diagnostic capabilities by enabling accurate and detailed assessments of blood cell morphology. These tools facilitate the early recognition of disorders, such as neutropenia, and support timely intervention and treatment. In addition, significant improvements in the management of postpartum hemorrhage have been achieved through the organization of multidisciplinary teams, adherence to evidence-based guidelines, and the incorporation of modern treatment protocols, all of which have contributed to better clinical outcomes in obstetric practice. Despite these advances, postpartum hemorrhage remains the leading cause of maternal mortality worldwide, highlighting the continued importance of progress in this field.

This book brings together the most recent advances in the diagnosis and management of hemoglobinopathies, the most common inherited blood disorders. By combining traditional approaches with cutting-edge innovations—including gene therapy, advanced diagnostics, nutritional support, and multidisciplinary care—remarkable progress has been achieved in improving both patient outcomes and quality of life.

Finally, I would like to extend my sincere gratitude to all contributors who participated in the preparation of this volume. In particular, my deepest thanks go to Kristina Kardum Cvitan, whose invaluable assistance greatly contributed to the successful completion of this work.

Silva Zupančić Šalek
Haematology Divisiopm,
Department of Internal Medicine,
Clinical Hlospital Sveti Duh,
Zagreb, Croatia

Section 1

Progress in Hemoglobinopathies

Chapter 1

Advances in Hemoglobinopathies: From Molecular Insights to Therapeutic Innovations

Behzad Davarnia and Sara Arish

Abstract

Hemoglobinopathies, such as thalassemia and sickle cell anemia, are among the most common genetic disorders worldwide, impacting more than 250,000 newborns annually. These inherited conditions arise from mutations in globin genes that cause abnormalities in the structure or synthesis of hemoglobin. While initially concentrated in tropical and subtropical regions, migration and demographic shifts have broadened their impact worldwide. Advances in the understanding of hemoglobin structure and gene regulation have elucidated mechanisms underlying these disorders, such as mutations affecting transcription, RNA splicing, and protein stability. Diagnostic strategies like hemoglobin electrophoresis, high-performance liquid chromatography (HPLC), and next-generation sequencing (NGS) have enhanced the detection and classification of hemoglobinopathies. Management approaches range from blood transfusions and iron chelation therapy to emerging genetic therapies, including gene editing with CRISPR-Cas9 and autologous stem cell transplantation. These innovations hold transformative potential, offering curative prospects for conditions previously managed symptomatically. Comprehensive screening and genetic counseling remain pivotal in reducing disease prevalence, especially in high-risk populations. This paper highlights the molecular basis, clinical variations, diagnostic advances, and therapeutic developments in hemoglobinopathies, emphasizing the global need for equitable access to innovative treatments.

Keywords: thalassemia, hemoglobinopathy, genetic disorders, hemoglobin, sickle cell disease

1. Introduction

Each year, over 250,000 newborns worldwide are born with a disorder in the structure or synthesis of hemoglobin (Hb), known as hemoglobinopathies. These disorders, which include conditions like thalassemia and sickle cell anemia, were originally more prevalent in tropical and subtropical regions. However, due to migration and social changes, these conditions have now spread globally and are a growing concern in many countries. According to statistics, the birth rate of children with these disorders is particularly high in certain regions. For instance, areas such as the Mediterranean, the Middle East, and South Asia have higher prevalence rates of thalassemia and sickle cell anemia (5–8 children per 1000 births), with birth rates of affected infants significantly above the global average. It is estimated that out of every 1000 births worldwide, two to three children are born with some form of hemoglobinopathy [1].

Sub-Saharan African countries, such as Nigeria, Ghana, and Cameroon, have the highest prevalence of sickle cell disease (SCD), with up to 40% of the population being carriers. The trait's persistence in these regions is linked to its protective role against malaria. Countries like Italy, Greece, Cyprus, and Turkey have high rates of beta-thalassemia, a common hemoglobinopathy in the region. Countries such as Saudi Arabia, Oman, and Iraq face a high prevalence of both sickle cell disease and thalassemia. The high rate of consanguineous marriages in these regions significantly contributes to the frequency of these disorders. Nations like India, Pakistan, Bangladesh, and Thailand are heavily affected by alpha- and beta-thalassemia. Additionally, certain tribal populations in India are particularly impacted by sickle cell disease. Due to the significant impact of these disorders, many countries have implemented genetic counseling and screening programs to reduce the birth rates of affected newborns and identify carriers. These programs are especially important in countries like the United Kingdom, the United States, Iran, and various countries in Southeast Asia, where identifying carriers and educating families can effectively reduce the transmission of these diseases to future generations. Moreover, this high birth rate of affected infants highlights the need for comprehensive healthcare, therapeutic, and educational strategies globally to mitigate the effects of these inherited diseases [2, 3].

2. Structure of hemoglobin

Hemoglobin (Hb) is a complex protein found in erythrocytes that plays a critical role in transporting oxygen throughout the body. Its structure comprises four subunits, each of which contains a heme group that binds to oxygen. Hemoglobin has a tetrameric structure, meaning it is composed of four protein subunits. Each hemoglobin molecule has two alpha (α) and two beta (β) chains in adult hemoglobin (HbA). These subunits work together to enable hemoglobin to efficiently bind and release oxygen [4].

Globin Gene Structure refers to the organization and sequence of the genes that encode the globin chains in hemoglobin. These genes are arranged in clusters and are highly conserved across different species.

Globin genes are primarily located within two main clusters on human chromosomes 11 and 16. These genes are arranged in a specific order and include regulatory elements that control their expression across various developmental stages. The two main types of globin genes are:

α-globin cluster (Chromosome 16): This contains two α-globin genes and is organized as α (α1 and α2) → ζ (embryonic). These genes are expressed early in embryonic development and throughout fetal and adult life, contributing to the formation of hemoglobin [5].

β-Globin cluster (Chromosome 11): This cluster encompasses the β-globin gene, which is responsible for synthesizing the β-globin chain of hemoglobin. Additionally, it contains the γ-globin genes responsible for producing fetal hemoglobin (HbF) during gestation, the δ-globin gene that contributes to the formation of HbA2, and the ε-globin gene involved in the synthesis of embryonic hemoglobin. The genes within the β-globin cluster are systematically organized in the 5′ to 3′ direction as follows: ε (embryonic) → γ (fetal) → δ (adult) → β (adult). During fetal development, the γ-globin genes, which encode fetal hemoglobin (HbF), are ultimately supplanted by the β-globin gene, which encodes adult hemoglobin (HbA) after birth. This specific arrangement facilitates a smooth transition from fetal to adult hemoglobin, as the γ-globin genes undergo silencing while the β-globin gene is activated following delivery [6].

Globin genes are expressed in a coordinated manner during various stages of human development. During embryonic development, the ζ and ε globin genes are primarily expressed. In fetal development, the γ-globin genes (γA and γG) are predominantly expressed, forming fetal hemoglobin (HbF). After birth, the γ-globin genes undergo silencing, while the β-globin gene is activated. This transition results in the production of adult hemoglobin (HbA), which consists of two α-globin chains and two β-globin chains. Understanding the precise location and sequence of globin genes is critical for elucidating the genetic basis of hemoglobinopathies. Mutations or deletions in these genes can result in disorders like sickle cell disease and thalassemia, which impact the structure or production of hemoglobin [7].

It is important to note that hemoglobinopathies (e.g., thalassemia and sickle cell disease) and clotting disorders (e.g., hemophilia) are both classified as inherited blood disorders, but they are fundamentally different in their genetic basis and physiological impact. While hemoglobinopathies are caused by mutations in the globin genes (on chromosomes 11 and 16), which impair oxygen transport, hemophilia results from mutations in clotting factor genes (e.g., F8 or F9 on the X chromosome), leading to defective blood clotting. Despite this distinction, both are often studied together in genetic research due to their shared classification as inherited hematological disorders and the overlap in diagnostic and management approaches, such as genetic counseling and prenatal screening.

Mutations in globin genes are specifically associated with conditions like sickle cell disease and thalassemia, while clotting factor deficiencies (like hemophilia), platelet disorders, and thrombophilia arise from defects in entirely different sets of genes involved in coagulation. Therefore, while these disorders are grouped together in the context of inherited blood diseases, they have no direct genetic or physiological link (**Figure 1**).

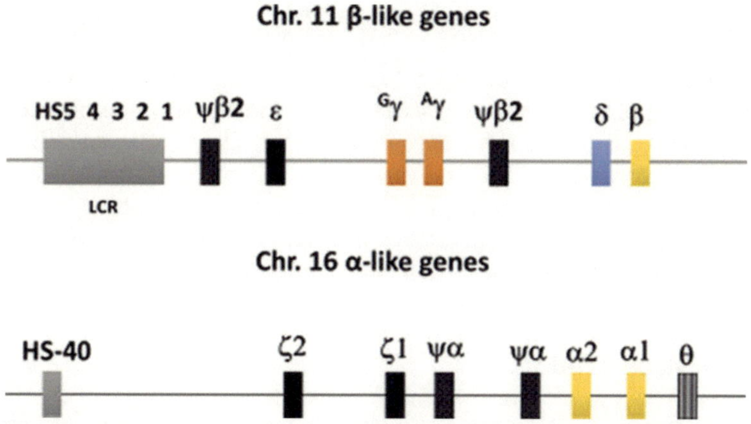

Figure 1.
Globin gene clusters: this schematic representation illustrates the β-like globin gene cluster located on chromosome 11 and the α-like globin gene cluster situated on chromosome 16. It depicts the organization of functional genes (e.g., β, γ, and α) alongside pseudogenes (e.g., ψβ2), as well as significant regulatory elements, including the locus control region (LCR) and HS-40, which are essential for the regulation of gene expression.

3. Protein analysis

In 1956, Vernon Ingram conducted an investigation into the structural components of human hemoglobin by fractionating its peptide products following digestion with the proteolytic enzyme trypsin, which specifically cleaves peptide chains at arginine and lysine residues. Ingram's analysis identified 30 distinct peptide fragments derived from human hemoglobin. Previous research has demonstrated that human hemoglobin is composed of approximately 580 amino acids, which include a total of 60 arginine and lysine residues. This finding suggests that hemoglobin consists of two identical polypeptide chains, with each chain containing 30 arginine and lysine residues [8].

Around the same time, reports emerged concerning a family whose members exhibited both HbS and Hb Hopkins II variants of hemoglobin. Some family members who carried both variants had offspring with either normal hemoglobin, single heterozygosity for one variant, or double heterozygosity for both variants, reflecting the genotypes of their parents. This pattern of inheritance provided early evidence that human hemoglobin production is influenced by at least two distinct genes. Shortly after these findings, researchers identified the amino-terminal amino acid sequence of human hemoglobin. This sequence showed an equal proportion of valine-leucine and valine-histidine, with two moles of each present per mole of hemoglobin. This discovery supported the hypothesis that human hemoglobin is a tetramer composed of two pairs of distinct polypeptide chains, known as the α- and β-globin chains. Subsequent investigations have revealed that hemoglobin (Hb) in normal adults consists of a minor fraction, comprising approximately 2–3% of the total hemoglobin, which exhibits distinct electrophoretic mobility compared to the predominant form. The primary component has been designated as HbA, while the less common component is identified as HbA2. Further research has demonstrated that HbA2 is a tetramer composed of two normal α chains and two polypeptide chains that closely resemble the β chain, referred to as delta (δ) chains [9].

4. Developmental expression of hemoglobin

The developmental expression of hemoglobin involves a sequence of changes in the types of hemoglobin synthesized by the body at various developmental stages, reflecting the evolving demands for oxygen transport. The regulation of hemoglobin expression is intricately controlled and varies across distinct fetal and postnatal phases. The principal forms of hemoglobin include fetal hemoglobin (HbF), adult hemoglobin (HbA), and smaller quantities of other variants, such as HbA2. The following provides a detailed description of the temporal progression of hemoglobin expression:

4.1 Fetal hemoglobin (HbF)

Expression: During fetal development, the predominant form of hemoglobin is fetal hemoglobin (HbF), which consists of two alpha (α) and two gamma (γ) globin chains, denoted as $\alpha 2\gamma 2$. This variant has a higher affinity for oxygen compared to adult hemoglobin, facilitating the efficient transfer of oxygen from the maternal bloodstream to the fetus through the placenta.

Regulation: HbF expression is regulated by the γ-globin gene, and its synthesis progressively decreases after birth. The high affinity of HbF for oxygen is essential for efficient oxygen transfer in the hypoxic environment of the womb.

Transition: During late fetal development and postnatally, γ-globin chains are replaced by β-globin chains, leading to the synthesis of adult hemoglobin [10].

4.2 Adult hemoglobin (HbA)

Expression: After birth, hemoglobin A (HbA) becomes the predominant form of hemoglobin. It is composed of two alpha (α) and two beta (β) globin chains, denoted

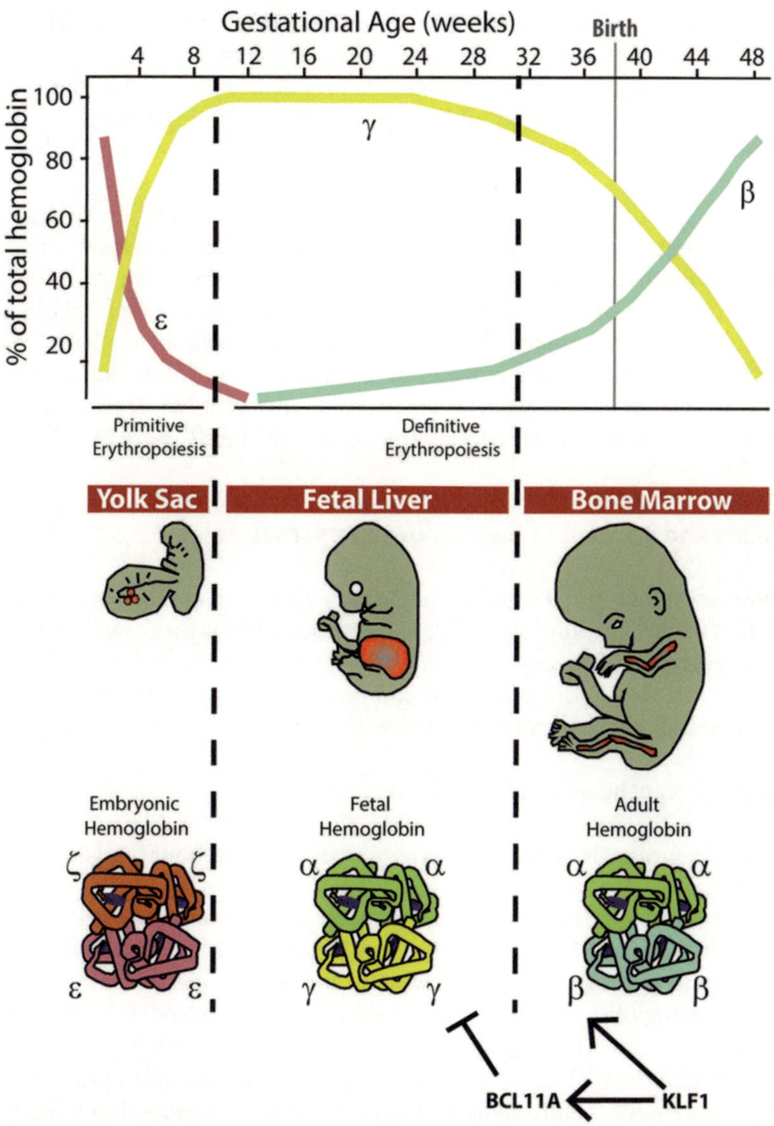

Figure 2.
Hemoglobin synthesis during development: Illustration of the developmental switch in hemoglobin synthesis, showing the transition from embryonic hemoglobin (ε and ζ chains) in the yolk sac to fetal hemoglobin (γ chains) in the fetal liver, and finally to adult hemoglobin (β chains) in the bone marrow.

as α2β2. Hemoglobin A has a lower affinity for oxygen compared to fetal hemoglobin (HbF), facilitating a more efficient release of oxygen to tissues in need.

Regulation: The transition from fetal hemoglobin (HbF) to adult hemoglobin (HbA) is a critical part of the biological process known as "hemoglobin switching," which involves changes in the expression of globin chain genes. After birth, the expression of the β-globin gene is initiated, leading to a reduction in HbF levels. By the end of the first year of life, HbA becomes the predominant form of hemoglobin [11].

4.3 HbA2

A minor component of adult hemoglobin is hemoglobin A2 (HbA2), which consists of two alpha (α) chains and two delta (δ) chains, denoted as α2δ2. In healthy adults, HbA2 accounts for approximately 2–3% of the total hemoglobin.

Regulation: The δ-globin gene, responsible for encoding the delta chain, exhibits lower expression levels compared to the β-globin gene. Although HbA2 is present in trace amounts in adults, its concentration remains relatively stable and does not experience significant variations after the neonatal period.

Abnormal regulation of hemoglobin switching can lead to disorders such as sickle cell disease and thalassemia, where the production of normal adult hemoglobin is disrupted. Some research aims to increase the expression of HbF in adults to alleviate the symptoms of these disorders, as HbF has a protective effect against the sickling of red blood cells in sickle cell disease. In summary, the development of hemoglobin involves a carefully regulated sequence of transitions from embryonic to fetal to adult forms. These changes are essential for meeting the oxygen requirements at different life stages, and any disruptions in this process may lead to various hemoglobinopathies (**Figure 2**) [12, 13].

5. Synthesis and control of hemoglobin expression

The synthesis and regulation of hemoglobin expression are intricately controlled processes that ensure the appropriate type of hemoglobin is produced during various stages of development. Hemoglobin consists of globin chains (α, β, γ, and δ) and heme groups, and the synthesis of these components is precisely coordinated to form functional hemoglobin molecules throughout different developmental stages.

5.1 Hemoglobin synthesis in development

Hemoglobin synthesis occurs in a series of stages throughout fetal and postnatal development:

Embryonic Hemoglobin: In the early stages of development, specifically during embryogenesis (weeks 3–12), hemoglobin synthesis is characterized by the production of embryonic hemoglobin (HbE), which consists of ζ and ε globin chains. This form of hemoglobin is critical for oxygen transport in the developing embryo; however, HbE is eventually replaced by fetal hemoglobin as development progresses.

Fetal Hemoglobin (HbF): As the fetus develops, γ-globin chains progressively replace ε-globin chains, resulting in the synthesis of fetal hemoglobin (HbF), which is composed of two α-globin chains and two γ-globin chains. HbF exhibits a higher affinity for oxygen, a critical characteristic that facilitates the transfer of oxygen from the mother to the fetus *via* the placenta. HbF remains the predominant form of hemoglobin in the fetal bloodstream until shortly after birth.

Adult Hemoglobin (HbA): Following birth, the synthesis of hemoglobin A (HbA) begins, consisting of two alpha-globin chains and two beta-globin chains. This process replaces fetal hemoglobin (HbF) as the predominant form of hemoglobin. Adult hemoglobin is specifically designed to facilitate the release of oxygen in tissues with the greatest demand for it.

HbA2: A small fraction of adult hemoglobin, referred to as HbA2, consists of two α-globin chains and two δ-globin chains. Typically, HbA2 constitutes approximately 2–3% of total hemoglobin and serves as a marker of normal globin gene expression [14–16].

5.2 Regulatory mechanisms of Hemoglobin synthesis

The regulation of hemoglobin gene expression is controlled at the transcriptional and post-transcriptional levels, primarily by developmentally regulated genes that activate different globin genes at different stages.

Locus Control Region (LCR): This critical regulatory element, located upstream of the β-globin gene cluster, is essential for modulating the expression of the β-globin gene family. The locus control region (LCR) interacts with specific transcription factors to enhance the expression of the β-globin and γ-globin genes during fetal development. In adulthood, the LCR plays a significant role in regulating the transition from fetal hemoglobin (HbF) to adult hemoglobin (HbA) after birth [17].

Transcription Factors: Several transcription factors regulate the expression of globin genes at various stages of development. For instance, GATA-1, NF-E2, and KLF1 are critical for activating the α-globin and β-globin genes. In contrast, BCL11A and SOX6 are implicated in the postnatal silencing of fetal hemoglobin genes.

Epigenetic Regulation: Modifications such as DNA methylation and changes in histone modifications play critical roles in regulating globin gene expression. These epigenetic factors are instrumental in mediating the silencing of fetal globin genes (γ-globin) while simultaneously facilitating the activation of adult globin genes (β-globin) [18].

5.3 Hemoglobinopathies and disorders

Hemoglobinopathies are genetic disorders that arise from mutations or structural alterations in the globin genes, resulting in the synthesis of abnormal hemoglobin. These conditions are predominantly inherited in an autosomal recessive pattern. Consequently, individuals with one defective allele (heterozygotes) act as carriers, whereas those with two defective alleles (homozygotes) manifest the disorder. Common hemoglobinopathies include sickle cell disease, thalassemia, and various platelet disorders, such as hemophilia and von Willebrand disease, as well as deficiencies in clotting factors and thrombophilia (**Table 1**).

5.4 Diagnosis and management of hemoglobinopathies

Diagnosis of hemoglobinopathies is often carried out through blood tests such as:

Hemoglobin electrophoresis: This technique separates different types of hemoglobin based on their electrical charge and is used to identify abnormal hemoglobin variants.

High-performance liquid chromatography (HPLC): This method quantifies the amount of different hemoglobin types in the blood.

Quantitative disorders of globin chain synthesis/accumulation	**Qualitative disorders of globin structure: structural variants of hemoglobin**
A. β-Thalassemia Clinical classification: β-Thalassemia minor or trait β-Thalassemia major β-Thalassemia intermedia Biochemical/genetic classification: β0-Thalassemia β+-Thalassemia δ-Thalassemia γ-Thalassemia Lepore fusion gene δβ-Thalassemia εγδβ-Thalassemia HPFH "Dominant" β-thalassemia (structural variants with β-thalassemia phenotype) β-Thalassemia with other variants: HbS/β-thalassemia HbE/β-thalassemia Other	A. Sickle cell disorders SA, sickle cell trait SS, sickle cell anemia/disease SC, HbSC disease S/β thal, sickle β-thalassemia disease S with other Hb variants: D, O-Arab, other SF, Hb S/HPFH
B. α-Thalassemia Deletions of α-globin genes: One gene: α+-thalassemia Two genes in cis: α0-thalassemia Two genes in trans: homozygous α+-thalassemia (phenotype of α0-thalassemia) Three genes: HbH disease Four genes: Hydrops fetalis with Hb Bart's Nondeletion mutants: Hb Constant Spring Other	B. Hemoglobins with decreased stability (unstable hemoglobin variants) Mutants causing congenital Heinz body hemolytic anemia Acquired instability—oxidant hemolysis: Drug-induced, G6PD deficiency
C. De novo and acquired α-thalassemia α-Thalassemia with mental retardation syndrome (ATR): Due to large deletions on chromosome 16 involving the α-globin genes Due to mutations of the ATRX transcription factor gene on chromosome X α-Thalassemia associated with myelodysplastic syndromes (ATMDS): Due to mutations of the ATRX gene	C. Hemoglobins with altered oxygen affinity High/increased oxygen affinity states: Fetal red cells Decreased RBC 2,3-BPG Carboxyhemoglobinemia, HbCO Structural variants Low/decreased oxygen affinity states: Increased RBC 2,3-BPG Structural variants
	D. Methemoglobinemia Congenital methemoglobinemia: Structural variants Cytochrome b5 reductase deficiency Acquired (toxic) methemoglobinemia
	E. Posttranslational modifications Nonenzymatic glycosylation Amino-terminal acetylation Amino-terminal carbamylation Deamidation

Table 1.
Classification of hemoglobin disorders.

DNA sequencing and mutation analysis: These tests identify the specific mutations in the globin genes that are responsible for the hemoglobinopathy.

Management of hemoglobinopathies may involve:

Blood transfusions to alleviate anemia and reduce complications such as stroke or organ damage.

Bone marrow or stem cell transplantation has the potential to offer a curative treatment for certain hemoglobinopathies, including sickle cell disease and β-thalassemia.

Gene therapy: Recent advancements in gene therapy demonstrate significant potential for treating hemoglobinopathies by correcting defective genes or enhancing fetal hemoglobin (HbF) expression.

Medications: Hydroxyurea is used to increase HbF production in individuals with sickle cell disease, which helps reduce the frequency of sickling events and related complications [19, 20].

6. Disorders of hemoglobin synthesis

Disorders of hemoglobin synthesis primarily result from defects in the production of the globin chains that compose the hemoglobin molecule. Hemoglobin, found in red blood cells, is essential for transporting oxygen throughout the bloodstream. Any defect in its synthesis results in imbalanced or ineffective oxygen transport, leading to anemia and other associated health complications. Hemoglobinopathies are genetic disorders arising from mutations or structural alterations in the globin genes, which result in abnormal hemoglobin production. These disorders are typically inherited in an autosomal recessive pattern. Individuals with one defective gene (heterozygotes) are carriers, whereas those with two defective genes (homozygotes) experience significant manifestations of the disorder. Common hemoglobinopathies include:

6.1 Thalassemias

Thalassemias are inherited hematologic disorders characterized by a partial or complete reduction in the synthesis of one or more globin chains. These disorders are classified based on the specific globin chain affected, resulting in two distinct forms: α-thalassemia and β-thalassemia.

6.1.1 α-Thalassemia

α-Thalassemia is a hereditary disorder resulting from mutations or deletions in the α-globin genes located on chromosome 16. Typically, individuals possess four copies of the α-globin gene, with two copies on each chromosome. The severity of α-thalassemia depends on the number of affected copies of the α-globin gene. These mutations predominantly manifest as gene deletions, which are more common, whereas point mutations are comparatively rare. Most cases of α-thalassemia are attributed to substantial deletions that remove one or more α-globin genes. This deletional α-thalassemia manifests in various forms, depending on the number of affected gene copies:

- Silent carrier silent carrier (−α/αα): Only one α-globin gene is deleted. Typically asymptomatic.

- α-Thalassemia trait (−α/−α or −−/αα): Two α-globin genes are deleted, either one from each chromosome (−α/−α) or both from one chromosome (−−/αα). Characterized by mild anemia, it frequently presents with no symptoms or only minimal symptoms.

- Hemoglobin H disease (−−/−α): Three α-globin genes are deleted, resulting in moderate to severe anemia. The remaining single α-globin gene is insufficient to produce an adequate quantity of α-chains to balance with the β-chains, which leads to the formation of hemoglobin H (HbH), an unstable hemoglobin composed of β-chain tetramers. Associated with moderate to severe anemia and splenomegaly, it often necessitates occasional blood transfusions.

- α-Thalassemia major (−−/−−): The deletion of all four α-globin genes results in a severe condition known as hydrops fetalis. In this condition, the absence of functional α-globin chains leads to the production of hemoglobin Bart's, which is composed of γ-chain tetramers. Hydrops fetalis is typically fatal either in utero or shortly after birth.

- Point mutations or small insertions and deletions: In rare instances, point mutations or small insertions and deletions within the α-globin gene or its regulatory regions may lead to non-deletional α-thalassemia. These mutations may have significant effects on gene expression, RNA processing, and protein stability. Mutations in regulatory regions can diminish the expression of the α-globin gene, resulting in inadequate production of α-globin. Furthermore, mutations that affect mRNA splicing can lead to the generation of unstable or ineffective α-globin mRNA, thereby decreasing the synthesis of functional α-globin chains. Certain point mutations may produce unstable α-globin proteins that undergo rapid degradation. A notable example of a non-deletional α-thalassemia mutation is the Hb Constant Spring mutation, characterized by a point mutation that extends the α-globin chain, rendering it unstable. Individuals with the Hb Constant Spring mutation typically exhibit a milder phenotype of hemoglobin H disease [21–23].

Clinical Manifestations: α-Thalassemia is characterized by anemia, ineffective erythropoiesis, and compensatory erythroid hyperplasia, resulting in the overproduction of red blood cell precursors. This condition arises from the absence or reduction of functional α-globin chains, leading to an imbalance between α- and β-globin chains and the subsequent formation of abnormal hemoglobin molecules. This imbalance precipitates ineffective erythropoiesis, hemolysis, and chronic anemia. In severe manifestations of the disease, such as hemoglobin H disease and hydrops fetalis, the deficiency of functional α-globin significantly impairs oxygen delivery and can be life-threatening. The management of α-thalassemia may require regular blood transfusions, particularly in cases of hemoglobin H disease. Additionally, for severe α-thalassemia, prenatal diagnosis and genetic counseling are essential for early detection and potential therapeutic interventions.

6.1.2 β-Thalassemia

β-Thalassemia is a genetic disorder resulting from mutations in the β-globin gene located on chromosome 11, leading to diminished or absent production of β-globin.

Each individual possesses two β-globin genes (one on each chromosome), meaning that these mutations can significantly reduce or completely inhibit β-globin chain synthesis. This imbalance has a consequential effect on the α-globin chains, ultimately resulting in ineffective erythropoiesis and hemolytic anemia. In contrast to α-thalassemia, which frequently involves large deletions, β-thalassemia is predominantly caused by point mutations, along with small insertions or deletions that impair the synthesis of β-globin. The types of β-thalassemia including:

β-Thalassemia minor (heterozygous): Beta-thalassemia minor is a benign hematological condition characterized by the presence of one normal allele of the beta-globin gene (e.g., B+/B or B0/B). Individuals diagnosed with thalassemia minor are typically asymptomatic; however, they may present with mild anemia. If both parents are carriers of the condition, there is a 25% probability with each pregnancy that their offspring will inherit homozygous thalassemia [24].

β-Thalassemia intermedia: Beta-thalassemia intermedia is situated within the clinical spectrum of beta-thalassemia and is characterized by a range of genetic variations that allow for partial production of beta chains (e.g., B+/B0 and B+/B+). Additionally, there are rare occurrences of simultaneous mutations affecting both beta and alpha-globin genes.

Individuals diagnosed with thalassemia intermedia typically present at a later stage compared to those with thalassemia major. Patients with thalassemia intermedia experience milder forms of anemia and, by definition, do not require regular blood transfusions; however, some may need transfusions on an occasional basis. Those at the more severe end of the clinical spectrum commonly present between the ages of 2 and 6 years. Although these individuals can survive without consistent blood transfusions, their growth and development may be adversely affected. Conversely, some patients may remain entirely asymptomatic until adulthood, experiencing only mild weakness. Generally, the signs and symptoms associated with thalassemia intermedia manifest during childhood or later [25].

β-Thalassemia major (Cooley's anemia):Beta-thalassemia is a significant clinical condition that arises when individuals are either homozygous or compound heterozygous for severe mutations in the beta-globin gene, exemplified by genotypes such as B+/B+, B+/B0, or B0/B0. The clinical manifestations associated with thalassemia major generally become evident between 6 months and 2 years of age. Affected children often present with severe anemia and failure to thrive, characterized by insufficient weight gain or growth relative to expected developmental milestones. Additionally, they may exhibit signs of jaundice, indicated by the yellowing of the skin and sclera, alongside notable pallor. These patients typically require frequent blood transfusions, which, if not adequately monitored, can lead to iron overload [26].

The genetic mutations associated with β-thalassemia generally impact multiple facets of gene function, including transcription, RNA splicing, mRNA stability, and translation:

Promoter mutations: Mutations within the β-globin promoter region reduce the transcriptional rate, leading to decreased levels of β-globin mRNA. These mutations are typically associated with β^+-thalassemia.

Splice site mutations: These mutations interfere with the normal splicing of the β-globin mRNA precursor, resulting in the production of abnormal or unstable mRNA, which in turn causes reduced β-globin synthesis. Certain splice site mutations may be responsible for β^+-thalassemia, while others can lead to β^0-thalassemia.

Nonsense mutations: Nonsense mutations generate premature stop codons, leading to the production of truncated and nonfunctional β-globin proteins. These mutations are the primary cause of β^0-thalassemia.

Frameshift mutations: Small insertions or deletions can alter the reading frame, leading to the synthesis of abnormal and often nonfunctional β-globin proteins. These frameshift mutations are commonly associated with β^0-thalassemia.

Mutations in untranslated regions (UTRs): Mutations occurring in the 5′ or 3' UTRs can destabilize the mRNA, thereby reducing β-globin synthesis and contributing to the development of β^+-thalassemia.

Symptoms of β-thalassemia include severe anemia, bone marrow expansion that results in skeletal abnormalities, and iron overload due to chronic transfusions, which may lead to organ damage, particularly affecting the heart and liver. Management strategies may involve blood transfusions, iron chelation therapy to prevent iron overload, and bone marrow or stem cell transplantation in cases of severe illness. Furthermore, advancements in gene therapy present promising avenues for future treatments of β-thalassemia by addressing the underlying genetic mutations [27].

6.1.3 Genetic counseling and prenatal diagnosis

The anticipation of beta-thalassemia depends on identifying carriers, providing genetic counseling, and implementing prenatal diagnosis. The literature extensively documents the processes involved in carrier identification. Genetic counseling informs individuals and at-risk couples, particularly those both identified as carriers, about the mode of inheritance, the genetic risks associated with having affected offspring, and the natural history of the disease, including available treatments and investigational therapies. Prenatal diagnosis for pregnancies identified as having an elevated risk of complications can be conducted through the analysis of fetal DNA derived from fetal cells obtained *via* amniocentesis, typically performed between 15 and 18 weeks of gestation, or through chorionic villus sampling at 11 weeks of gestation. Prior to the implementation of prenatal testing, it is crucial to identify both alleles associated with the specific condition. Presently, researchers are investigating the potential of analyzing fetal DNA in maternal plasma and fetal cells in maternal blood to identify paternal mutations. Families with established disease-causing mutations may qualify for preimplantation genetic diagnosis.

Prenatal diagnosis (PND), genetic counseling, carrier screening, and the option to terminate an affected fetus are critical components in the prevention of thalassemia. This comprehensive approach is not only cost-effective but has also significantly reduced the prevalence of thalassemia in various countries. To facilitate efficient and timely prenatal diagnosis and genetic counseling, it is imperative to understand the range and distribution of thalassemia mutations within specific populations. Such knowledge is essential for the effective and prompt implementation of these services [28].

6.2 Hereditary persistence of fetal hemoglobin (HPFH)

HPFH is a condition in which fetal hemoglobin (HbF), normally replaced by adult hemoglobin after birth, continues to be produced into adulthood. While this condition is typically asymptomatic, it can provide partial compensation for reduced or absent adult hemoglobin in individuals with thalassemia or sickle cell disease, resulting in milder clinical manifestations. Hereditary persistence of fetal hemoglobin

(HPFH) is associated with mutations in the regulatory regions of the γ-globin genes, which lead to the continued expression of these genes beyond the neonatal period. Although HPFH is generally considered benign, its presence in individuals with other hemoglobinopathies—such as sickle cell disease or β-thalassemia—can improve clinical outcomes by mitigating symptoms through the prevention of red blood cell sickling or the reduction of anemia severity.

Disorders of hemoglobin synthesis result in an imbalance of globin chains, disrupting the structure and stability of red blood cells. This leads to several pathological conditions:

Hemolytic anemia: Characterized by the increased destruction of abnormal or ineffective red blood cells.

Bone marrow hyperplasia: The bone marrow expands in an attempt to produce a greater number of red blood cells, which may result in skeletal deformities.

Iron overload: Frequent blood transfusions can lead to an accumulation of iron, potentially causing damage to various organs if left untreated.

Management strategies include regular blood transfusions, iron chelation therapy to reduce iron overload, and, in severe cases, bone marrow transplantation. Furthermore, gene therapy and innovative genetic editing techniques are currently being investigated as potential curative interventions for these disorders [29, 30].

7. Disorders of hemoglobin structure

Structural abnormalities in hemoglobin arise from mutations in the globin genes, leading to changes in the protein's amino acid sequence. These alterations can impair hemoglobin's ability to bind oxygen or destabilize its structure.

7.1 Sickle cell disease

Sickle cell disease (SCD) is a hereditary hematological disorder characterized by the presence of an abnormal form of hemoglobin known as hemoglobin S (HbS). In individuals affected by SCD, red blood cells, which are typically round and flexible, become deformed and assume a rigid, crescent or sickle-like shape under conditions of reduced oxygen tension. These sickle-shaped erythrocytes can obstruct blood flow, leading to a range of health complications. Sickle cell disease is inherited in an autosomal recessive manner, requiring that an individual acquire two copies of the sickle cell gene—one from each parent—to manifest the disease phenotype. If only one copy of the gene is inherited, the individual is classified as a carrier, known as having sickle cell trait, and typically exhibits no clinical symptoms. Nonetheless, carriers can still transmit the gene to their offspring. Sickle cell disease is more prevalent among individuals of African, Mediterranean, Middle Eastern, and Indian descent. The World Health Organization (WHO) reports that approximately 300,000 infants are born with sickle cell disease annually worldwide. It is estimated that 20 million individuals are affected by this condition, with the highest prevalence observed in sub-Saharan Africa, certain regions of India, and the Middle East. Sickle cell disease is a genetic disorder caused by a mutation in the β-globin gene, which encodes a subunit of hemoglobin. This mutation leads to the substitution of the amino acid glutamic acid with valine at position 6 of the β-globin chain. Consequently, this alteration leads to the formation of hemoglobin S (HbS), which polymerizes under low oxygen conditions, resulting in the deformation of red blood cells into a sickle shape and a subsequent loss of their normal elasticity. Sickle cell disease is diagnosed through a blood test known as hemoglobin electrophoresis, which can identify the presence of abnormal hemoglobin. Newborn screening for sickle cell disease has become standard practice in many countries, facilitating early diagnosis and intervention. A characteristic symptom of sickle cell disease (SCD) is the occurrence of painful episodes known as vaso-occlusive crises. During these episodes, sickled red blood cells impede blood flow to various organs and tissues, resulting in significant pain in areas such as the chest, back, joints, and abdomen. Sickled red blood cells exhibit increased fragility and a higher propensity for hemolysis compared to normal red blood cells, contributing to the chronic condition of anemia. This anemia is characterized by symptoms such as fatigue, weakness, and dyspnea. Individuals diagnosed with SCD face an elevated risk of infections due to compromised splenic function. The spleen, an organ essential for the immune response, is often damaged by the sickling of red blood cells, which impairs its ability to filter pathogens. Furthermore, the occlusion of cerebral blood vessels may result in cerebrovascular accidents, particularly in pediatric patients with SCD. Prolonged obstruction of blood flow can induce ischemic damage to critical organs, including the kidneys, liver, lungs, and heart. Such damage may lead to severe complications, including renal failure and pulmonary hypertension [31, 32].

7.2 Sickle cell disease (HbS)

Sickle cell disease is caused by a point mutation in the β-globin gene, in which glutamic acid at position 6 is substituted with valine. This singular alteration results in the aggregation of hemoglobin molecules, leading to the formation of rigid, sickle-shaped erythrocytes that have difficulty traversing blood vessels. The deformation of these cells causes occlusions in blood flow, which can lead to pain, anemia, and potential organ damage. Sickle cell disease is among the most thoroughly investigated and recognized hemoglobinopathies in the field of hematology.

7.3 Hemoglobin C disease (HbC)

Hemoglobin C disease is a hemoglobinopathy resulting from a mutation in the β-globin gene, specifically characterized by the substitution of lysine for glutamic acid at position 6. This alteration leads to the synthesis of abnormal hemoglobin molecules. In contrast to sickle cell disease, hemoglobin C does not cause the sickling of red blood cells; nevertheless, it may still contribute to the development of mild hemolytic anemia.

7.4 Hemoglobin E disease

Hemoglobin E is a variant of hemoglobin resulting from a mutation in the β-globin gene, specifically characterized by the substitution of lysine for glutamic acid at position 26. This variant is particularly prevalent in Southeast Asia and is associated with mild anemia. However, when hemoglobin E coexists with β-thalassemia, it can lead to more severe clinical complications [33].

8. Other hereditary blood disorder

Among other hereditary blood disorders, this condition can be attributed to deficiencies in clotting factors, hemophilia, platelet disorders, thrombophilia, and von Willebrand disease. Hemophilia, a rare disorder characterized by the inability of blood to clot properly due to a deficiency of blood-clotting proteins, will be elucidated.

8.1 Types of Hemophilia

Hemophilia affects approximately 1 in 5000 male births worldwide. Hemophilia A is the most prevalent form, accounting for 80–85% of cases, while hemophilia B constitutes approximately 15–20%. It is estimated that around 400,000 individuals globally are living with hemophilia. This rare, inherited bleeding disorder is characterized by deficiencies in clotting factors, which are essential proteins for normal blood coagulation. In males (XY), having a single X chromosome means that a mutation in either the F8 or F9 gene results in the manifestation of hemophilia. In females (XX), individuals are generally asymptomatic carriers, as the normal allele on the second X chromosome compensates for the mutated allele. However, approximately 10–20% of carriers may present with mild symptoms due to skewed X-inactivation, in which the X chromosome containing the normal gene is preferentially inactivated. The two primary types of hemophilia are hemophilia A, which is caused by a deficiency in clotting factor VIII, and hemophilia B, which results from a deficiency in clotting factor IX. Both types are classified as X-linked recessive disorders, predominantly affecting males, while females are generally asymptomatic carriers. Hemophilia is characterized by prolonged blooding, episodes of spontaneous hemorrhage, and internal bleeding, particularly affecting the joints (hemarthrosis) and muscles, which can lead to significant pain, swelling, and long-term joint damage. In severe cases, this condition can precipitate life-threatening hemorrhages. The classification of hemophilia is determined by the levels of clotting factors, categorizing the disease into severe, moderate, or mild forms:

Severe: Characterized by factor activity levels of less than 1%, this classification is associated with frequent spontaneous bleeding episodes. Patients often experience spontaneous bleeding, including hemarthrosis (bleeding into joints), as well as bleeding into muscles and internal organs, even in the absence of injury.

Moderate Hemophilia: Defined by factor activity levels ranging from 1–5%, this classification results in bleeding episodes that typically follow minor trauma. Bleeding is observed after minor injuries or surgical interventions.

Mild Hemophilia: Identified by factor activity levels between 5% and 40%, this classification is characterized by bleeding that generally occurs only in response to injury or surgical procedures. Patients with mild hemophilia primarily experience bleeding during significant trauma or invasive medical interventions.

Complications associated with hemophilia can result in chronic joint damage, anemia, and an increased susceptibility to infections due to recurrent bleeding episodes. Patients diagnosed with severe forms of the disorder typically require lifelong management to effectively mitigate these complications. Hemophilia A is caused by mutations in the F8 gene located on the X chromosome, which encodes coagulation factor VIII. Notably, common mutations include intron 22 inversions, which account for approximately 45–50% of severe cases, along with point mutations and deletions. Conversely, hemophilia B arises from mutations in the F9 gene, also located on the X chromosome, which encodes factor IX. These mutations encompass a variety of alterations, including missense and nonsense mutations, as well as small insertions and deletions [34–36].

9. Antenatal and newborn hemoglobinopathy screening

Antenatal and newborn hemoglobinopathy screening is a critical public health initiative designed to identify carriers and individuals affected by hemoglobinopathies, including sickle cell disease (SCD) and thalassemias, either during pregnancy or shortly after birth. This proactive approach is instrumental in preventing severe health complications, facilitating timely medical interventions, and providing genetic counseling to at-risk families.

9.1 Antenatal screening

Detect carriers of hemoglobinopathies (e.g., sickle cell trait and β-thalassemia trait) among expectant parents. Identify pregnancies at risk of resulting in offspring with severe hemoglobinopathies. A complete blood count (CBC) assists in identifying anemia or abnormal red blood cell indices (e.g., low mean corpuscular volume [MCV]). Hemoglobin Electrophoresis facilitates the detection of abnormal hemoglobin variants, such as HbS, HbC, or HbE. DNA Analysis serves to confirm specific genetic mutations in high-risk cases. Genetic Counseling is essential when both parents are carriers of a hemoglobinopathy, as there is a 25% probability that their child will inherit a severe disorder. In this context, parents are provided with information regarding reproductive options, including prenatal diagnostic techniques (chorionic villus sampling or amniocentesis) and preimplantation genetic testing [37].

9.2 Newborn screening

Newborn screening represents a comprehensive system designed to identify, treat, manage, and potentially eradicate genetic disorders from the neonatal stage. A primary advantage of newborn screening programs is their ability to enhance health outcomes for patients who receive early diagnoses and appropriate interventions. Nevertheless, several challenges persist, including the occurrence of false positives and false negatives. Fortunately, the implementation of innovative molecular technologies for confirmatory testing has effectively addressed these concerns. Early detection of infants affected by hemoglobinopathies, such as sickle cell disease (SCD) or severe thalassemias, is crucial. It is essential to initiate early interventions to prevent complications, including infections, stroke, and organ damage. The dried blood spot test involves analyzing a small blood sample obtained *via* a heel prick using techniques such as isoelectric focusing (IEF), which separates hemoglobin types based on their electrical charge. High-performance liquid chromatography (HPLC), which quantifies different hemoglobin variants. DNA testing is used in ambiguous cases or to confirm results [19].

9.3. Next-generation sequencing (NGS): NGS has significantly enhanced the precision of molecular diagnostics for thalassemias due to advancements in dosage mutation tests that identify large deletions or duplications, as well as the implementation of multiple gene panel tests utilizing massively parallel sequencing. These technologies have not only improved diagnostic accuracy but have also deepened our understanding of the genomic mechanisms underlying this condition.

In NGS-based diagnostics, the methodology involves the massively parallel sequencing of clonally amplified DNA molecules, which requires substantial computational resources and specialized software for effective data analysis. This approach can be applied to the entire genome, the exome, or specific targeted regions of the genome. A critical component of NGS is the design of the probe set for DNA capture, which necessitates a high degree of homology among genes in the alpha and beta clusters. While NGS is proficient in detecting single nucleotide substitutions, insertions, and small deletions, it has limitations in accurately identifying other forms of genomic variations [38].

9.3 Impact of screening

Reduces morbidity and mortality associated with hemoglobinopathies. Facilitates the prevention of affected children being born through informed reproductive choices. Screening programs are extensively implemented in areas with a high prevalence of hemoglobinopathies, including sub-Saharan Africa, South Asia, the Middle East, and Mediterranean countries. In high-resource nations (e.g., the United States and the United Kingdom), universal newborn screening protocols ensure prompt diagnosis and effective management. In regions with established screening programs, the incidence of severe complications resulting from hemoglobinopathies has markedly declined. In the United Kingdom, approximately 300 infants with sickle cell disease are identified annually through newborn screening initiatives [39].

10. New perspectives of treatment in Hemoglobinopathies

Hemoglobinopathies, which include sickle cell disease (SCD) and thalassemia, constitute a group of inherited hematological disorders associated with significant morbidity and mortality. Traditional treatment modalities primarily focus on symptom management and the prevention of associated complications; however, recent advancements in therapeutic approaches are presenting promising prospects for more definitive, long-term interventions. These innovative strategies encompass genetic therapies, novel pharmacologic agents, and improvements in bone marrow transplantation techniques. Genetic treatments for hemoglobinopathies, such as sickle cell disease (SCD) and thalassemia, are among the most promising approaches for potentially curing these inherited blood disorders. These therapies aim to modify the patient's genetic material to rectify the underlying mutations that cause the disease. Genetic treatments include gene therapy, gene editing, and genetic modification of stem cells.

10.1 Gene therapy

Gene therapy encompasses the introduction, removal, or modification of genetic material within a patient's cells to treat or prevent disease. Specifically, in the context of hemoglobinopathies, the objective of gene therapy is to either introduce a functional copy of the hemoglobin gene or rectify the mutations that underlie the condition. Hematopoietic stem cells (HSCs) are harvested from the patient's bone marrow or peripheral blood [40].

Stem cells are genetically modified in a laboratory setting using viral vectors, predominantly lentiviral vectors, to incorporate a normal, functional copy of the gene responsible for hemoglobin production, specifically the β-globin gene. Following modification, the stem cells are reintroduced into the patient's body, facilitating the production of healthy red blood cells that contain normal hemoglobin.

Goal: The primary objective of this approach is to achieve a cure for the disease by correcting the defective gene within the patient's own cells, thereby facilitating the production of normal hemoglobin and eliminating the need for blood transfusions or other interventions.

A notable success in this field is the application of LentiGlobin in the treatment of β-thalassemia, which has resulted in patients no longer requiring blood transfusions post-treatment. In the case of sickle cell disease (SCD), gene therapy has shown the ability to enhance the production of fetal hemoglobin (HbF), reducing the sickling of red blood cells and alleviating the symptoms associated with the disease. The challenges of this method include high costs, technical complexities, long-term safety concerns, and issues of accessibility and affordability, particularly in low-resource settings [41].

In numerous clinical trials, researchers have employed autologous hematopoietic stem cell transplantation, in which a patient's own stem cells are modified to correct the sickle cell mutation or enhance HbF production. Notably, LentiGlobin, a gene therapy that uses a lentiviral vector to introduce a modified copy of the β-globin gene into the patient's stem cells, has demonstrated promising outcomes.

Key Trials: In a 2016 trial, a patient diagnosed with severe sickle cell disease (SCD) who received gene-modified stem cells *via* LentiGlobin was able to stop regular blood transfusions. Post-treatment, the patient exhibited no clinical symptoms of sickle cell disease, as their hematologic profile reflected the production of normal hemoglobin [42].

10.2 Gene editing

Gene editing represents a more direct approach compared to traditional gene therapy. It employs techniques such as CRISPR-Cas9 to facilitate precise alterations to the genomes of a patient's cells. The objective of gene editing in the context of hemoglobinopathies is to directly rectify mutations within the globin genes or alter the expression of genes that may compensate for dysfunctional hemoglobin. A transformative tool for achieving this goal is the CRISPR-Cas9 system, which can be engineered to target specific DNA sequences with precision. This system employs guide RNA to direct the Cas9 nuclease to a designated locus in the genome, where it induces a double-strand break. Subsequently, the cellular repair mechanisms address this break, allowing researchers to insert or delete genetic material or correct mutations. In the case of sickle cell disease, CRISPR-Cas9 is employed to edit the β-globin gene in stem cells with the intent to:

- Correct the mutation responsible for sickling, or
- Reactivate fetal hemoglobin (HbF) production. HbF exhibits a higher affinity for oxygen and does not undergo sickling in the same manner as adult hemoglobin. The reactivation of HbF is one of the most promising strategies for mitigating sickle cell crises.

In the context of thalassemia, similar strategies can be implemented to correct mutations in the β-globin gene that cause the disease or to modify gene expression to enhance the production of normal hemoglobin. While CRISPR-Cas9 has demonstrated promising outcomes in early-stage trials, challenges persist, including off-target effects (where the enzyme makes unintended edits), the efficiency of gene editing, and the long-term safety of these modifications. Nonetheless, the ability to directly modify DNA at the genetic level holds significant potential for providing a permanent cure.

Case success: In 2019, CRISPR-based gene editing was successfully performed on two patients with sickle cell disease (SCD), resulting in a substantial increase in hemoglobin F (HbF) levels. Both patients were able to discontinue blood transfusions, and their disease symptoms were significantly reduced or eliminated. The CRISPR-Cas9 methodology aims to reactivate the HbF gene, which is typically silenced after birth, to mitigate the severity of sickling. The efficacy of this technique was demonstrated in clinical trials conducted by Editas Medicine, which indicated that gene-edited cells produced elevated levels of HbF, leading to improved clinical outcomes [43, 44].

In 2024, the UK achieved a significant milestone in treating beta-thalassemia with the approval of Casgevy, a CRISPR-based gene therapy. This treatment, developed by Vertex Pharmaceuticals in collaboration with CRISPR Therapeutics, is now available through the NHS for patients over 12 years old who have transfusion-dependent beta-thalassemia (TDT) and meet specific criteria. The therapy uses CRISPR technology to edit the patient's hematopoietic stem cells, correcting the defective gene responsible for the disorder. After the edited cells are reintroduced, the body can produce functional hemoglobin, potentially eliminating the need for lifelong blood transfusions. This therapy is considered groundbreaking due to its curative potential and is administered as a one-time treatment following a preparatory chemotherapy regimen to replace the patient's dysfunctional stem cells. Clinical trials have shown remarkable results, with the majority of patients achieving independence from regular blood transfusions. This development is a beacon of hope for individuals with beta-thalassemia, particularly those without access to compatible bone marrow donors.

11. Clinical success

Early-stage clinical trials have shown that genetic therapies, especially gene therapy and gene editing, can significantly reduce the severity of hemoglobinopathies and may even offer potential cures. For example, in sickle cell disease, trials involving gene-modified stem cells suggest that patients can maintain a good quality of life without regular transfusions and experience fewer sickle cell crises. Similarly, in thalassemia, patients who have received gene-modified stem cell transplantation have demonstrated a marked decrease in their dependence on blood transfusions.

Challenges: Cost and Accessibility: Gene therapy and gene editing treatments are associated with high costs, and access to these advanced therapies may be limited, particularly in low-resource settings.

Long-Term Safety: Although initial results are promising, the long-term effects of gene therapies, including potential cancer risk or unintended genetic alterations, remain a considerable concern.

Efficiency: The efficacy of gene therapies and editing techniques can vary, prompting researchers to investigate methods for enhancing the effectiveness of these processes [45].

12. Future prospects

Future treatment strategies for hemoglobinopathies may involve integrating gene therapy, gene editing, and genetically modified stem cells to offer a more effective and lasting cure. As technological advancements progress, it is imperative to prioritize the affordability and accessibility of these therapies, particularly in countries with a high prevalence of hemoglobinopathies. Researchers are actively investigating novel methodologies to address other genetic blood disorders using similar approaches, which could potentially broaden the range of conditions amenable to treatment through gene therapies.

13. Clinical variation of the hemoglobinopathies

The considerable mutational diversity associated with β-thalassemia often leads to the classification of individuals as compound heterozygotes, indicating the presence of different variants within their β-globin genes. This genetic variability creates a broad spectrum of clinical severity, including intermediate forms known as thalassemia intermedia, which require fewer blood transfusions. In certain geographical regions, the prevalence of hemoglobinopathies is notably high, resulting in a common occurrence of individuals with two distinct hemoglobin disorders.

Historically, accurate diagnoses posed significant challenges; however, advancements in DNA sequencing technologies have substantially improved the clarity of these cases. For example, individuals who are heterozygous for both HbS and β-thalassemia can now be precisely identified as compound heterozygotes. Specific genetic combinations may lead to previously unexplained milder forms of what would typically be classified as severe hemoglobinopathies. For instance, when an individual is homozygous for β-thalassemia and has lost one or two α-globin genes, the clinical symptoms are frequently less severe. This phenomenon is attributable to a decreased imbalance in globin chain production. Similarly, individuals who are homozygous for either β-thalassemia or sickle cell disease and possess a hereditary persistence of fetal hemoglobin (HPFH) variant may experience a reduction in the severity of their condition. This attenuation in severity can be ascribed to the increased production of

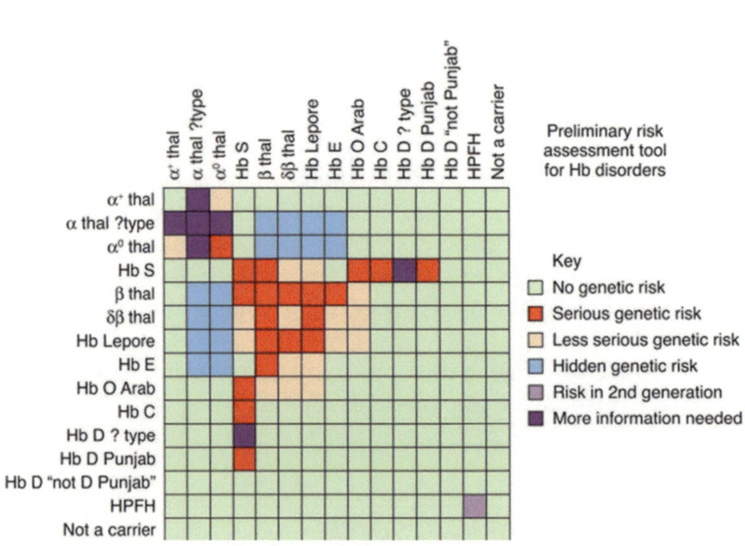

Figure 3.
A hemoglobinopathy tool that outlines the expected clinical severity associated with various homozygous or compound heterozygous genotypes.

γ-globin chains, which can effectively compensate for the inadequate production of β-globin chains [4, 46].

The relative severity of various homozygous and compound heterozygous hemoglobinopathies is concisely summarized in a risk assessment tool developed by the National Health Service's Sickle Cell and Thalassemia Screening Programme.

Figure 3 presents a comprehensive risk assessment tool for hemoglobinopathies, designed to predict the clinical severity associated with different genetic combinations, including homozygous and compound heterozygous states. The chart systematically evaluates the genetic risks arising from various hemoglobin variants, such as α-thalassemia, β-thalassemia, Hb S (sickle cell hemoglobin), Hb C, Hb D, and other less common hemoglobinopathies. Each intersection in the grid represents the clinical risk associated with a specific combination of these genetic variants. The color-coded matrix provides a clear and intuitive risk categorization: white cells indicate no genetic risk, red cells signify serious risks with potentially severe clinical outcomes, blue cells represent milder or hidden risks, purple cells highlight risks that may manifest in subsequent generations, and gray cells denote cases where further information is required to assess risk accurately. This tool is particularly valuable in genetic counseling, assisting clinicians in identifying high-risk combinations, guiding carrier screening, and informing reproductive decision-making. By visualizing potential risks, this tool serves as a practical resource for managing hemoglobinopathies, especially in regions where such disorders are prevalent. It facilitates early intervention and planning, ultimately contributing to improved healthcare outcomes for affected individuals and their families.

Author details

Behzad Davarnia* and Sara Arish
Medical Genetics and Pathology, Ardabil University of Medical Sciences, Ardabil, Iran

*Address all correspondence to: b.davarnia@gmail.com

References

[1] Tuo Y, Li Y, Li Y, Ma J, Yang X, Wu S, et al. Global, regional, and national burden of thalassemia, 1990-2021: A systematic analysis for the global burden of disease study 2021. Eclinicalmedicine. 2024;**72**

[2] Modell B, Darlison M. Global epidemiology of haemoglobin disorders and derived service indicators. Bulletin of the World Health Organization. 2008;**86**(6):480-487

[3] Lippi G, Mattiuzzi C. Updated worldwide epidemiology of inherited erythrocyte disorders. Acta Haematologica. 2020;**143**(3):196-203

[4] Emery AE, Rimoin DL, editors. Principles and Practice of Medical Genetics. Vol. 2. Churchill Livingstone; 2021

[5] Hua-bing Z, De-Pei L, Chih-Chuan L. The control of expression of the α-globin gene cluster. International Journal of Hematology. 2002;**76**:420-426

[6] Moleirinho A, Seixas S, Lopes AM, Bento C, Prata MJ, Amorim A. Evolutionary constraints in the β-globin cluster: The signature of purifying selection at the δ-globin (HBD) locus and its role in developmental gene regulation. Genome Biology and Evolution. 2013;**5**(3):559-571

[7] Lu HY, Orkin SH, Sankaran VG. Fetal hemoglobin regulation in beta-thalassemia. Hematology/Oncology Clinics of North America. 2023;**37**(2):301-312

[8] Ingram VM. A specific chemical difference between the globins of normal human and sickle-cell anaemia haemoglobin. Nature. 1956;**178**(4537):792-794

[9] Ahmed SG, Ibrahim UA. Non-s sickling hemoglobin variants: Historical, genetic, diagnostic, and clinical perspectives. Oman Medical Journal. 2021;**36**(3):e261

[10] Manca L, Masala B. Disorders of the synthesis of human fetal hemoglobin. IUBMB Life. 2008;**60**(2):94-111

[11] Sankaran VG, Orkin SH. The switch from fetal to adult hemoglobin. Cold Spring Harbor Perspectives in Medicine. 2013;**3**(1):a011643

[12] Ivaldi G, Barberio G, Harteveld CL, Giordano PC. HbA2 measurements in β-thalassemia and in other conditions. Thalassemia Reports. 2014;**4**(2):1832

[13] Higgins TN, Khajuria A, Mack M. Quantification of HbA2 in patients with and without β-thalassemia and in the presence of HbS, HbC, HbE, and HbD Punjab hemoglobin variants: Comparison of two systems. American Journal of Clinical Pathology. 2009;**131**(3):357-362

[14] Zakaria M, Hassan T, Sherief L, Erhabor O. Thalassemia Syndromes: New Insights and Transfusion Modalities. BoD–Books on Demand; 2023. pp. 3-29

[15] Thein SL. Molecular basis of β thalassemia and potential therapeutic targets. Blood Cells, Molecules & Diseases. 2018;**70**:54-65. DOI: 10.1016/j.Bcmd.2017.06.001

[16] Needs T, Gonzalez-Mosquera LF, Lynch DT. Beta Thalassemia. In: StatPearls. Treasure Island. FL: StatPearls Publishing; 2022

[17] Li Q, Peterson KR, Fang X, Stamatoyannopoulos G. Locus control regions. Blood, The Journal of the

American Society of Hematology. 2002;**100**(9):3077-3086

[18] Bauer DE, Kamran SC, Orkin SH. Reawakening fetal hemoglobin: Prospects for new therapies for the β-globin disorders. Blood, The Journal of the American Society of Hematology. 2012;**120**(15):2945-2953

[19] Ghosh K, Colah R, Manglani M, Choudhry VP, Verma I, Madan N, et al. Guidelines for screening, diagnosis and management of hemoglobinopathies. Indian Journal of Human Genetics. 2014;**20**(2):101

[20] Kutlar F. Diagnostic approach to hemoglobinopathies. Hemoglobin. 2007;**31**(2):243-250

[21] Vichinsky EP. Clinical manifestations of α-thalassemia. Cold Spring Harbor Perspectives in Medicine. 2013;**3**(5):a011742

[22] Piel FB, Weatherall DJ. The α-Thalassemias. New England Journal of Medicine. 2014;**371**(20):1908-1916

[23] Yamsri S, Sanchaisuriya K, Fucharoen G, Sae-Ung N, Fucharoen S. Genotype and phenotype characterizations in a large cohort of β-thalassemia heterozygote with different forms of α-thalassemia in Northeast Thailand. Blood Cells, Molecules & Diseases. 2011;**47**(2):120-124

[24] Origa R. Beta-Thalassemia. In: Adam MP, Ardinger HH, Pagon RA, Wallace SE, Bean LJH, Stephens K, Amemiya A, editors. GeneReviews® [Internet]. Seattle; 1993-2020. Seattle (WA): University of Washington; 2020. Available from: http://www.ncbi.nlm.nih.gov/books/NBK1426/CitationonPubMed

[25] Akhavan-Niaki H, Derakhshandeh-Peykar P, Banihashemi A, Mostafazadeh A, Asghari B, Ahmadifard MR, et al. A comprehensive molecular characterization of beta thalassemia in a highly heterogeneous population. Blood Cells, Molecules & Diseases. 2011;**47**(1):29-32

[26] Rund D, Rachmilewitz E. Beta-thalassemia. The New England Journal of Medicine. 2005;**353**(11):1135-1146

[27] Peixeiro I, Silva AL, Romão L. Control of human β-globin mRNA stability and its impact on beta-thalassemia phenotype. Haematologica. 2011;**96**(6):905

[28] Mensah C, Sheth S. Optimal strategies for carrier screening and prenatal diagnosis of α-and β-thalassemia. Hematology. 2021;**2021**(1):607-613

[29] Amato A, Cappabianca MP, Perri M, Zaghis I, Grisanti P, Ponzini D, et al. Interpreting elevated fetal hemoglobin in pathology and health at the basic laboratory level: New and known γ-gene mutations associated with hereditary persistence of fetal hemoglobin. International Journal of Laboratory Hematology. 2014;**36**(1):13-19

[30] Forget BG. Molecular basis of hereditary persistence of fetal hemoglobin. Annals of the New York Academy of Sciences. 1998;**850**(1):38-44

[31] Ware RE, de Montalembert M, Tshilolo L, Abboud MR. Sickle cell disease. The Lancet. 2017;**390**(10091): 311-323

[32] Rees DC, Williams TN, Gladwin MT. Sickle-cell disease. The Lancet. 2010;**376**(9757):2018-2031

[33] Kato GJ, Piel FB, Reid CD, Gaston MH, Ohene-Frempong K, Krishnamurti L, et al. Sickle cell disease.

Nature Reviews Disease Primers. 2018;**4**(1):1-22

[34] Srivastava A, Brewer AK, Mauser-Bunschoten EP, Key NS, Kitchen S, Llinas A, et al. Guidelines for the management of hemophilia. Haemophilia. 2013;**19**(1):e1-e47

[35] Zimmerman B, Valentino LA. Hemophilia: In review. Pediatrics in Review. 2013;**34**(7):289-295

[36] Srivastava A, Santagostino E, Dougall A, Kitchen S, Sutherland M, Pipe SW, et al. WFH guidelines for the management of hemophilia. Haemophilia. 2020;**26**:1-158

[37] Ghosh K, Ghosh K, Agrawal R, Nadkarni AH. Recent advances in screening and diagnosis of hemoglobinopathy. Expert Review of Hematology. 2020;**13**(1):13-21

[38] Achour A, Koopmann TT, Baas F, Harteveld CL. The evolving role of next-generation sequencing in screening and diagnosis of hemoglobinopathies. Frontiers in Physiology. 2021;**12**:686689

[39] Goonasekera HW, Paththinige CS, Dissanayake VHW. Population screening for hemoglobinopathies. Annual Review of Genomics and Human Genetics. 2018;**19**(1):355-380

[40] Goodman MA, Malik P. The potential of gene therapy approaches for the treatment of hemoglobinopathies: Achievements and challenges. Therapeutic Advances in Hematology. 2016;**7**(5):302-315

[41] Christakopoulos GE, Telange R, Yen J, Weiss MJ. Gene therapy and gene editing for β-thalassemia. Hematology/Oncology Clinics of North America. 2023;**37**(2):433-447

[42] Kumar H, Sharma V, Wadhwa SS, Gowda DM, Kaushik S, Joseph AM, et al. LentiGlobin administration to sickle cell disease patients: Effect on serum markers and vaso-occlusive crisis. Cureus. 2024;**16**(1)

[43] Frangoul H, Altshuler D, Cappellini MD, Chen YS, Domm J, Eustace BK, et al. CRISPR-Cas9 gene editing for sickle cell disease and β-thalassemia. New England Journal of Medicine. 2021;**384**(3):252-260

[44] Fu B, Liao J, Chen S, Li W, Wang Q, Hu J, et al. CRISPR–Cas9-mediated gene editing of the BCL11A enhancer for pediatric β0/β0 transfusion-dependent β-thalassemia. Nature Medicine. 2022;**28**(8):1573-1580

[45] Malik P. Gene therapy for hemoglobinopathies: Tremendous successes and remaining caveats. Molecular Therapy. 2016;**24**(4):668-670

[46] Shiva Raj KC, Basnet S, Gyawali P. Prevalence of hemoglobinopathies and hemoglobin variants. Nepal Medical College Journal. 2017;**19**(3):121-126

Chapter 2

Perspective Chapter: Recent Developments in the Diagnosis of Sickle Cell Disease

Mohammed AW. Almorish

Abstract

Sickle cell disease (SCD) is a prevalent disorder resulting from a beta-globin gene mutation, causing the production of abnormal hemoglobin known as hemoglobin S. The disease can manifest with sickled cells, leading to hemolysis, anemia, painful episodes, organ damage, and potentially death. The timely identification of SCD is pivotal in diminishing mortality rates and facilitating effective disease management. Consequently, a variety of methodologies have been formulated to identify SCD and carrier states with elevated sensitivity and specificity. These methodologies encompass screening assessments such as complete blood count, peripheral blood smears, and the sickling test; confirmatory evaluations like hemoglobin separation techniques; and genetic examinations, which tend to be costlier and require execution in centralized laboratories by highly trained professionals. Nevertheless, innovative portable point-of-care (POC) methodologies have been established to offer an economical, straightforward, and user-friendly apparatus for the detection of SCD. Examples include the integration of solubility tests with portable devices, the application of smartphone microscopic classifications, image processing techniques, rapid immunoassays, and sensor-based platforms. This chapter elucidates the existing and new emerging strategies for the identification of SCD and underscores the various potential approaches that could be utilized to assist in the prompt diagnosis of SCD.

Keywords: sickle cell disease (SCD), point-of-care (POC) tests, HPLC, lateral flow immunoassays, DNA microarrays, flow cytometry

1. Introduction

Sickle cell disease (SCD) is a hereditary condition resulting from a genetic mutation affecting hemoglobin production and leading to sickle hemoglobin formation. This disease, inherited in an autosomal recessive pattern, can present as SCD when combined with another hemoglobin S (HbS) gene or other hemoglobin abnormalities [1]. Individuals with SCD face organ damage, with an average lifespan 20 years lower than the general population. SCD affects around 300,000 newborns annually, primarily in countries like Nigeria, India, and the Democratic Republic of Congo, as well as regions like the Mediterranean and the Middle East, with migrations and historical events like the trans-Atlantic slave trade contributing to its spread. In the US, approximately 100,000 people are impacted by SCD [2, 3].

The pathophysiology of HbS involves the formation of long chains of hemoglobin due to low oxygen levels, leading to distorted red blood cells with heightened adhesion molecules [4]. This process results in rapid destruction of sickled cells, triggering an inflammatory response that contributes to acute and chronic damage in various organs, causing unpredictable complications such as vaso-occlusion and tissue damage [5]. Complications in SCD vary in severity and frequency depending on genetic factors like globin production variants, with heterozygous individuals typically experiencing issues later in life compared to homozygous individuals [4].

Newborns in countries with screening programs may receive early diagnoses through advanced assays such as high-performance liquid chromatography (HPLC), which detect hemoglobin variants and are verified via hemoglobin electrophoresis [6]. However, disparities in screening practices, particularly in nations where testing is optional, can result in missed diagnoses of SCD, compounded by the time-intensive nature of these methodologies and potential lapses in communication with parents [2]. These methodologies are inherently time-consuming, require sophisticated technological apparatus and/or considerable personnel training, and necessitate subsequent visits for result communication; thus, some confirmed SCD diagnoses may not be communicated to parents [7]. Solubility testing functions as a qualitative screening method for detecting HbS in capillary blood from individuals as young as 6 months; nevertheless, it is unable to distinguish between SCD and sickle cell trait and may present false negatives in patients with α-thalassemia trait and severe anemia, as well as false positives in cases of increased serum viscosity, erythrocytosis, and leukocytosis [8].

Emerging POC testing technologies, characterized by their accessibility, affordability, swift processing, and precision, are essential for ensuring effective communication of results to families and facilitating follow-up care for SCD patients, especially in at-risk communities. SCD may also be identified through normocytic anemia assessments, severe pain evaluations in emergencies, or prenatal testing, but the specific diagnostic rates via these methods remain unspecified [9].

Recent developments in the diagnosis of SCD have focused on leveraging advanced technologies to overcome the limitations of traditional diagnostic methods. These innovations aim to enhance accuracy, reduce costs, and improve accessibility, particularly in resource-limited settings. The integration of artificial intelligence, novel spectroscopic techniques, and mass spectrometry are at the forefront of these advancements, offering promising solutions for early and precise detection of SCD [10].

2. Recent advancements in diagnosis of SCD

A multitude of techniques and assessments are utilized for the identification and surveillance of SCD, classified into conventional diagnostic approaches and novel research-oriented methodologies, emphasizing recent advancements in the diagnostic processes for SCD.

2.1 Conventional diagnostic techniques in SCD

SCD can be prevented and diagnosed prenatally or in newborns through screening. Early diagnosis is crucial for initiating treatments that mitigate life-threatening complications and manage disease effectively. Diagnosis of SCD involves complete blood tests, blood smears, hemoglobin electrophoresis, HPLC, and genetic sickling tests. The hemoglobin S solubility assay and sodium metabisulfite test are applicable for individuals aged 6 months and older. Pregnant women should undergo screening ideally before 10 weeks of gestation. Recent studies have explored emerging portable techniques for early detection and diagnosis of SCD and carrier states [11, 12]. More comprehensive molecular genetic diagnostic tests are also accessible [13].

2.1.1 Hemoglobin electrophoresis

Hemoglobin electrophoresis is a critical diagnostic tool for SCD, offering valuable insights into the hemoglobin variants present in patients. This method is traditionally used to differentiate between normal hemoglobin (HbA) and HbS, as well as other variants such as hemoglobin C (HbC) and fetal hemoglobin (HbF) [14, 15].

Recent advancements have enhanced the utility of hemoglobin electrophoresis in diagnosing and managing SCD. For instance, it can help distinguish between severe delayed hemolytic transfusion reactions (DHTR) and hyperhemolysis syndrome in patients with SCD. The absence of HbA on electrophoresis can indicate DHTR, which is crucial for appropriate management and reducing morbidity and mortality [16]. Moreover, the development of POC technologies, such as the Gazelle-Multispectral microchip, has made hemoglobin electrophoresis more accessible, especially in low-resource settings. This technology allows for rapid and accurate newborn screening by detecting low concentrations of Hb variants, which is essential for early intervention and reducing SCD mortality [15]. While traditional electrophoresis methods have limitations in sensitivity and specificity, they remain a cornerstone in SCD diagnosis. However, novel approaches like mass spectrometry offer more sensitive and quantitative assessments, potentially improving diagnostic accuracy and patient monitoring, especially in the context of gene therapy trials [14]. In summary, hemoglobin electrophoresis remains a vital diagnostic tool for SCD, with recent innovations enhancing its applicability and accuracy. These advancements facilitate better disease management and early intervention, particularly in resource-limited settings, thereby improving patient outcomes.

2.1.2 Isoelectric focusing

Isoelectric focusing (IEF) is a classical laboratory method used in the diagnosis of SCD and other hemoglobinopathies, particularly in newborn screening programs. IEF is employed to separate hemoglobin variants based on their isoelectric points, allowing for the identification of abnormal hemoglobin such as HbS, which is responsible for SCD [1, 17]. This method is often used in conjunction with other techniques like HPLC and capillary electrophoresis to ensure accurate diagnosis [1].

The use of IEF in diagnosing SCD is well-established, particularly for early detection in newborns, which is crucial for preventing complications associated with the disease. IEF is typically performed alongside other confirmatory tests, such as the solubility test or electrophoresis on agar gel, to verify the presence of HbS [17]. This comprehensive approach helps in distinguishing between sickle cell trait and more severe forms of the disease, such as sickle cell anemia, which require different management strategies [17]. This method efficiently detects various types of hemoglobin like HbS and HbA in a short time, making it ideal for newborn screening despite being costly and requiring skilled staff due to the complexity of interpreting results and multiple bands present. Furthermore, IEF is advantageous as it only requires a small amount of sample and can be performed using dried blood spots [18]. While IEF remains a cornerstone in the diagnosis of SCD, it is important to consider the integration of newer technologies and methods that offer improved accuracy and efficiency. The combination of IEF with advanced techniques like capillary IEF and HPLC can provide a more comprehensive diagnostic framework, ensuring early and precise detection of SCD and related hemoglobinopathies [1].

2.1.3 High performance liquid chromatography

HPLC effectively separates hemoglobin fractions due to their differential interactions with the stationary phase, with each variant exhibiting a unique retention time [19]. It is instrumental in detecting various hemoglobin types, including HbF, Hb A2, HbS, and HbC, and offers superior sensitivity compared to electrophoresis, albeit with limitations in distinguishing variants sharing similar retention times [20]. Consequently, while HPLC is advantageous for monitoring patient conditions, it should not be utilized as a standalone diagnostic tool and must be corroborated with molecular analyses for accurate diagnosis [21]. HPLC demonstrates superior sensitivity in the separation of hemoglobin variants compared to electrophoresis.

2.1.4 Polymerase chain reaction methodologies

The genetic analysis is crucial for accurately identifying different forms of SCD by identifying mutations in the β-globin gene responsible for its development [22].

Polymerase chain reaction (PCR) is a potent diagnostic tool that utilizes enzymes to amplify specific genetic material segments. This process involves denaturation, annealing, and elongation, repeated over 20–40 thermal cycles [23]. PCR can identify single or multiple genes in a single tube through techniques like gel electrophoresis or sequencing. PCR-based methods like high-resolution melting (HRM) analysis are characterized by their simplicity, sensitivity, and cost-effectiveness, making them suitable for extensive screening of SCD genotypes and allele-specific amplification (ASA) along with a hot start system to achieve more precise single-tube genotyping, with the point mutation associated with sickle cell anemia serving as the model for single nucleotide polymorphisms (SNPs). HRM and ASA have enhanced prenatal and neonatal diagnostics [22, 24]. The amplification-refractory mutation system [ARMS] is another simple PCR technique for detecting mutations, particularly useful in prenatal diagnosis for sickle cell mutations. The ARMS technique has predominantly been utilized in prenatal diagnostics, particularly in the detection of sickle cell mutations within fetal samples. The sensitivity of ARMS has been evaluated by comparing results with the identification of hemoglobin variants through HPLC [25]. An allele-specific oligonucleotide hybridization method was introduced for sickle cell mutation detection, using fluorescent labels to differentiate allelic variations efficiently [26].

Recent innovations in PCR techniques have markedly improved the diagnostic capacity for SCD, providing expedited, economical, and readily available alternatives, especially beneficial in resource-constrained environments where conventional diagnostic approaches are impractical.

2.1.5 Restriction fragment length polymorphism

Restriction fragment length polymorphism (RFLP) is employed for the identification of SCD through restriction enzymes that eliminate the recognition site at the mutated βs gene. MstII, an early identified restriction enzyme, cuts DNA at the CCTNAGG sequence, and if thymine replaces adenine, the MstII restrictase recognition site is lost. The presence of mutations is indicated by the number of resulting bands following enzyme cleavage, with different band patterns observed in individuals with healthy (βA βA), sickle cell trait (βAβS), and sickle cell anemia homozygous (βSβS) genotypes [27]. Another enzyme used in sickle cell detection is Ddel I, which produces varying band lengths depending on the presence of the sickle cell anemia mutation [28, 29]. While RFLP remains a reliable method for SCD diagnosis, other techniques such as allele-specific recombinase polymerase amplification (RPA) and surface plasmon resonance (SPR) biosensors have also been developed. RPA offers rapid, low-cost testing with high sensitivity and specificity, suitable for point-of-care settings [26].

2.1.6 DNA microarrays and sequencing methodologies

DNA microarrays are arrays with immobilized DNA spots where hybridization events occur to indicate nucleic acid concentrations. They are used in genome-wide association studies to detect SNPs and copy number variants [25]. A recent study developed a comprehensive database integrating gene expression and genome-wide association studies data to examine the transcriptomic profiles associated with SCD [30]. Next-generation sequencing is utilized for mutation identification through whole-exome sequencing (WES) or whole-genome sequencing (WGS), aiding in predicting SCD severity and progression [31]. WES is specifically used to identify SNVs in the β-globin gene, providing a detailed description of the gene. Various studies have utilized these methods to uncover genetic modifications related to SCD severity, such as mutations in GOLGB1, ENPP1, SALL2, MBL2, and KLRC3, with WGS contributing to the Sickle Genome Project and the identification of genetic modifiers like BCL11A, HBB, UGT1A1, and APOL1 for precision medicine advancements [32, 33].

These developments focus on identifying differentially expressed genes and potential biomarkers that can aid in the diagnosis and management of SCD. The integration of microarray data with other genomic analyses has provided deeper insights into the molecular mechanisms underlying SCD, offering new avenues for diagnosis and treatment.

2.2 Novel and innovative approaches for the diagnosis of SCD

2.2.1 Image processing methodologies

Recent advancements in image processing techniques have significantly enhanced the detection and classification of SCD through various novel methodologies. These techniques primarily leverage deep learning and machine learning models to improve diagnostic accuracy and efficiency. One innovative approach combines conventional classifiers with segmented images and convolutional neural networks to automate SCD classification. This method achieves a high accuracy of 96.80% by integrating segmented images with CNN features and support vector machine (SVM) classifiers, offering a computationally efficient solution for medical image analysis [34]. Another study introduces a semi-automated system using digital microscopy to capture blood smear images, which are then processed using deep learning models like Darknet-19 and ResNet variants. This system demonstrates strong performance, achieving an average accuracy of around 97%, and is particularly beneficial for use in resource-limited settings [35].

Further advancements include the use of adaptive thresholding and contour-based segmentation methods for automatic SCD detection. This technique employs geometric feature extraction and applies them to classifiers such as ANN and SVM, achieving a maximum accuracy of 99.2% with SVM [36]. Additionally, a novel methodology utilizing watershed segmentation and region property analysis, such as centroid calculation, aids in the detection and counting of sickle cells, providing a valuable decision support system for medical experts [37]. Moreover, a deep learning approach using an improved wrapper-based feature selection technique with the InceptionV3 model has been proposed. This method extracts deep features from blood smear images and uses Multi-Objective Binary Gray Wolf Optimization for feature selection, enhancing classification accuracy to 96% with SVM [38].

These novel image processing techniques collectively demonstrate significant potential in improving the early diagnosis and management of SCD, offering high accuracy and efficiency while addressing the challenges of computational overhead and resource limitations. The integration of these methods into clinical practice could greatly benefit pathologists, especially in areas with limited access to specialized medical resources.

2.2.2 Flow cytometry methodologies

Recent advancements in flow cytometry have improved diagnostic capabilities for SCD, particularly in understanding its pathophysiology and predicting outcomes. The quantitative flow cytometry (qFC) method enables accurate quantification of HbF in red blood cells (RBCs). This technique provides a precise evaluation of the percentage of protected RBCs [%pRBC], with HbF content exceeding 10 pg./RBC, essential for preventing sickling and mutant HbS polymerization [1]. The qFC method exhibits a strong correlation with hematimetric indices and outperforms classical flow cytometry in predicting high-risk SCD patients, indicated by a higher area under the ROC curve [39]. Additionally, a no-lysis flow cytometry protocol has been established to characterize heterotypic aggregates of RBCs, leukocytes, and platelets in SCD, minimizing artifacts from traditional lysis methods for a more accurate thrombo-inflammatory phenotype representation. Significant increases in platelet-leukocyte aggregates and RBC-leukocyte aggregates were found in SCD, underscoring the role of RBCs in aggregate formation and the method's potential in elucidating systemic thrombo-inflammatory mechanisms in SCD [40].

Emerging functional microfluidic assays provide direct biomarkers of thromboinflammation, such as abnormal cell adhesion and aggregation, which are pivotal in SCD pathogenesis, thereby offering a viable approach for personalized risk assessment and therapeutic decision-making [41]. Imaging flow cytometry enhances diagnostic capabilities by integrating flow cytometry with microscopy for rapid, automated erythrocyte morphology and surface marker analysis in SCD, enabling the identification and quantification of RBC subpopulations indicative of disease severity and progression [42]. Moreover, flow cytometry's role in HbF measurement is evolving under new *in vitro* diagnostics regulations, emphasizing the necessity for accurate and rapid testing for personalized SCD management, given the significant variability in HbF distribution among patients affecting therapeutic outcomes. Accurate individual RBC HbF measurement is critical for optimizing treatment regimens and enhancing patient prognoses [43].

Advanced flow cytometry techniques, including imaging flow cytometry, have been developed to detect sickle cells based on cell morphology and population analysis. The flow cytometry assay developed by Beers et al. distinguishes sickle from normal RBCs based on morphology with high sensitivity and specificity. Another method, *in-vitro* photoacoustic flow cytometry developed by Cai et al., employs photothermal and photoacoustic spectra to detect hemoglobin S in sickle cells, facilitating the observation of sickling conditions [44, 45].

Microfluidic flow cytometry, as described by Liua et al., employs electrical impedance spectroscopy to identify shape modifications in normal versus sickled cells under hypoxic conditions. These innovative cytometric techniques demonstrate potential for evaluating sickling propensity in sickle cell anemia patients, yet further investigation is essential to assess their efficacy in disease severity monitoring and differentiating sickle cell trait from SCD [46].

Overall, the integration of advanced flow cytometry techniques in SCD diagnosis and management offers significant improvements in precision, speed, and clinical relevance, making it a promising tool for enhancing patient care [47].

2.2.3 Mechanical deformability of sickle cell approaches

Recent advancements in techniques for detecting the mechanical deformability of sickle cells have focused on microfluidics and mathematical modeling approaches. The Microfluidic Impedance Red Cell Assay (MIRCA) is a notable technique that mimics the capillary microvasculature environment, allowing for the measurement of RBC deformability by calculating the occlusion index. This index reflects the percentage of occlusion in the microfluidic chip, providing insights into the mechanical stress experienced by RBCs in SCD [48]. MIRCA is advantageous due to its low cost, portability, and ease of use compared to traditional methods like ektacytometry, making it suitable for routine clinical use and in low-resource settings [48]. Mathematical modeling has also been employed to analyze the flow of sickle RBCs in microvessels. These models use lubrication theory to simulate the rheological properties of sickle cells, providing insights into the pathogenesis of vaso-occlusion. The models demonstrate that decreased cell deformability leads to reduced axial velocity and increased adhesion to capillary walls, contributing to vaso-occlusion events [49, 50]. These findings align with experimental results and suggest potential for designing microfluidics-based diagnostic tools for SCD [50]. Additionally, a microfluidic platform has been developed to measure RBC deformability and oxygen saturation simultaneously. This platform reveals that polymer-containing RBCs exhibit decreased deformability, which is independent of oxygen levels, highlighting their role in SCD pathologies [51]. While these techniques offer promising avenues for detecting sickle cell deformability, they also present limitations. For instance, the MIRCA's reliance on impedance measurements may not fully capture the complexity of RBC deformability under varying physiological conditions. Moreover, while mathematical models provide valuable insights, they require validation through experimental data to ensure accuracy and applicability in clinical settings. Overall, these techniques represent significant progress in understanding and diagnosing SCD by focusing on the mechanical properties of sickle cells, with potential implications for therapeutic interventions and improved patient outcomes.

2.2.4 Lateral flow immunoassays

Recent advancements in lateral flow immunoassays (LFIA) have significantly enhanced the diagnosis of SCD, particularly in resource-limited settings. The development of a multiplexed, allele-specific recombinase polymerase amplification assay with lateral flow readout has been optimized for detecting multiple pathologic point mutations in the β-globin gene, which are responsible for most cases of SCD. This method offers a promising approach for rapid and accurate diagnosis [52]. The integration of optical nanoparticles (NPs) in LFIA has further improved diagnostic capabilities. These NPs, with their unique optical properties, serve as probes that enhance the sensitivity and specificity of LFIAs, making them a major tool in disease diagnostics [53]. This technological advancement is crucial for the effective management of SCD, especially in low- and middle-income countries (LMICs) where traditional diagnostic methods are often too costly and resource-intensive [54]. A novel E-junction lateral flow immunoassay has been specifically designed for widespread SCD screening in LMICs. This device is low-cost, point-of-care, and capable of diagnosing healthy individuals, those with SCD, and those with sickle cell trait using just a single drop of whole blood. The device's affordability, usability, and reliability make it suitable for implementation in these regions, addressing the high mortality rates associated with SCD due to limited access to diagnostics [4]. Additionally, the Sickle SCAN™ POC device has demonstrated high sensitivity and specificity for detecting hemoglobin variants HbA, HbS, and HbC. It is effective with both liquid blood and dried blood spots, even in samples with high HbF concentrations. This robustness and accuracy make it an excellent candidate for large-scale screening and diagnosis in resource-limited settings [55]. The HemoTypeSC™ test is a POC test and a valuable tool for the early diagnosis of SCD, particularly in resource-constrained environments. Its high sensitivity and specificity, along with the potential for using DBS, make it a practical option for large-scale screening initiatives. However, confirmatory testing with secondary methods is recommended to ensure diagnostic accuracy, especially in cases where resources allow [56, 57].

Recent innovations in LFIA, particularly those incorporating optical nanoparticles and novel device designs, have significantly improved the diagnosis of SCD. These advancements offer practical solutions for effective screening and management of SCD in both high-resource and low-resource environments, potentially reducing the disease's global burden.

2.2.5 Density-based separation methods

Recent advancements in density-based separation techniques have shown promise in the diagnosis of SCD. These methods leverage the distinct density properties of RBCs affected by SCD, which are denser than normal RBCs due to the presence of HbS. One innovative approach involves the use of microfluidic magnetic levitation, as demonstrated by Goreke et al. This method, known as MagDense, can detect minute density differences in individual RBCs, allowing for the identification of subpopulations within blood samples. The technique effectively distinguishes between HbS-containing RBCs and HbA-containing RBCs by measuring their levitation height in a paramagnetic medium. This method not only provides a high-resolution analysis of RBC density but also introduces the concept of "RBC levitational density width" as a measure of density dispersion, which correlates with clinical parameters like reticulocyte count and RBC distribution width [58]. Another promising technique is the use of aqueous multiphase systems (AMPS), which create step-gradients in density to separate RBCs. This method, as described by Kumar et al., allows for the rapid and visual identification of SCD by detecting dense cells characteristic of the disease. AMPS can differentiate between homozygous (Hb SS) and heterozygous (Hb SC) forms of SCD with high sensitivity and specificity, making it a viable POC diagnostic tool, especially in low-resource settings [59, 60]. Field evaluations of AMPS in Zambia have demonstrated its potential as a low-cost, accessible diagnostic method. Despite some challenges, such as false positives due to clotting and batch variations, the system has shown good sensitivity, particularly in young children, and is considered user-friendly by healthcare workers [61]. Overall, density-based separation techniques, including MagDense and AMPS, offer promising avenues for the diagnosis of SCD, providing rapid, accurate, and cost-effective solutions that could significantly improve disease management, especially in resource-limited areas.

2.2.6 Paper-based hemoglobin solubility methods

Recent advancements in paper-based hemoglobin solubility tests have shown promise in the diagnosis of SCD, particularly in resource-limited settings. The traditional sickle cell solubility test, or "sickle prep," is highly sensitive (99.9%) and specific (99.9%) for detecting HbS but can yield false negatives in patients with severe anemia or high levels of hemoglobin F, especially when HbS levels fall below 15% [62]. This limitation is significant in patients undergoing red cell exchange, where the sensitivity drops to 84% [62]. In contrast, a paper-based screening test evaluated by Kumar et al. demonstrated 100% sensitivity and specificity in identifying HbS, with a slight reduction in sensitivity (97.7%) when differentiating between sickle cell trait and disease [61]. This test's stability and longevity, particularly when stored at 4°C, make it a viable option for community-based screening programs, offering a low-cost, rapid, and accurate POC solution [61]. The assessment of the durability of paper-based screening tests indicates their stability for up to 180 days at 4°C, demonstrating 100% sensitivity and specificity for HbS detection and 97.7% sensitivity for distinguishing sickle cell trait from disease, making them suitable for community screenings in developing nations [63].

Furthermore, the HemeChip, a paper-based microchip electrophoresis platform, has shown high accuracy in identifying hemoglobin variants, including HbS, with 100% sensitivity and an overall diagnostic accuracy of 98.4% [64]. This technology is particularly beneficial in low-resource settings, providing an affordable and easy-to-use method for early diagnosis, which is crucial for reducing morbidity and mortality associated with hemoglobin disorders [64]. While non-invasive spectrophotometric methods for hemoglobin measurement have been explored, they tend to overestimate lab Hb concentrations and have lower sensitivity compared to traditional methods [65]. Additionally, the incorporation of machine learning using AutoML-based approach with UV-Vis absorbance spectroscopy significantly improves the accuracy of these tests, achieving 100% sensitivity and 93.84% specificity, thereby enhancing their utility as cost-effective diagnostic tools for sickle cell disease and trait in mass screening initiatives [66].

Therefore, while these methods offer some advantages, they are not yet as reliable as the paper-based tests for diagnosing SCD. Overall, paper-based hemoglobin solubility tests, particularly those using microchip electrophoresis, offer a promising alternative for SCD diagnosis, especially in settings where traditional laboratory resources are limited. These tests provide high sensitivity and specificity, making them suitable for widespread screening and early intervention in affected populations [61, 64].

2.2.7 Fluorescence-based optofluidic resonator

Recent innovations in fluorescence-based optofluidic resonators indicate their utility in diagnosing SCD. Research by Dai et al. investigates a waveguide optofluidic resonator for precise, real-time fluorescent assessments, particularly examining the interactions of Fe^{2+} and Fe^{3+} with protoporphyrin IX in a PBS medium. The findings reveal that the fluorescent signature of Fe^{2+} aligns with normal hemoglobin, contrasting with Fe^{3+}, which corresponds to SCD-associated hemoglobin, suggesting a possible pathogenic role of Fe^{3+} substitution [67]. Additionally, remote blood hemoglobin monitoring using hyperspectral color truthing has been developed to provide non-invasive, telemedicine-based assessments of blood hemoglobin levels, which are critical for SCD management [68]. For instance, near-infrared spectroscopy (NIRS) has been explored for monitoring tissue hemodynamics in SCD patients, showing sensitivity to differences in oxygenation and blood flow between SCD patients and healthy controls [69].

In summary, the fluorescence-based optofluidic resonator signifies a valuable diagnostic instrument for SCD, augmenting non-invasive techniques such as NIRS and hyperspectral imaging, thereby necessitating additional investigation to substantiate and incorporate these methodologies into clinical applications.

2.2.8 Sensors based on electrical impedance signal

Recent advancements in sensors based on electrical impedance signals have shown promising potential in the diagnosis and monitoring of SCD. These sensors leverage the unique electrical properties of sickle cells to provide diagnostic insights. One approach involves the use of bioimpedance sensing in microfluidic devices to analyze sickled RBCs of varying densities. This method can discriminate between low- and high-density sickle erythrocytes by measuring transit time, blockade amplitude, and phase shift of electrical signals as cells pass through microfluidic constrictions. This technique not only distinguishes between different RBC subpopulations but also offers a promising tool for monitoring therapeutic strategies in SCD and other red cell disorders [70]. Another innovative method employs an impedimetric CRISPR-dCas9-based biosensor system. This system is designed to detect the specific mutation responsible for sickle cell anemia. By using electrochemical impedance spectroscopy, this biosensor can quickly and cost-effectively identify the mutation, offering a linear measurement range between 40 and 1000 pM. The biosensor's rapid measurement time of 100 seconds makes it a valuable tool for efficient diagnosis [71]. Additionally, electrical impedance detection has been applied to monitor sickle cell vaso-occlusion in microfluidic capillary structures. This technique observes changes in resistance and reactance of sickle blood flow, which are indicative of progressive occlusion events, a hallmark of SCD [70]. Furthermore, dielectric spectroscopy has been used to study the dielectric properties of sickle cells under normoxic and hypoxic conditions. This method reveals changes in cell permittivity and conductivity, which can serve as diagnostic biomarkers for SCD. The technique's ability to rapidly analyze small sample volumes makes it suitable for clinical applications [72]. Overall, these electrical impedance-based methods provide valuable diagnostic capabilities for SCD, offering rapid, sensitive, and non-invasive options for disease detection and monitoring. Each approach has its unique advantages, contributing to a comprehensive toolkit for managing SCD.

2.2.9 Quartz crystal microbalance technology

Quartz Crystal Microbalance (QCM) technology has shown significant promise in the field of medical diagnostics, including the potential for diagnosing SCD. QCM is a highly sensitive, label-free biosensing technology that detects mass changes on a sensor surface, making it suitable for identifying disease biomarkers and other clinically relevant analytes [73]. Recent advancements in QCM biosensors have focused on enhancing their sensitivity and specificity through the integration of aptamers and molecular imprinting techniques. Aptamers, which are synthetic oligonucleotides or peptides, serve as biorecognition elements that can bind specifically to target molecules, including disease biomarkers. This specificity is crucial for the accurate detection of biomarkers associated with diseases like SCD [74]. The use of aptamer-based QCM biosensors has been highlighted for their ability to provide quick, stable, and sensitive detection, which is essential for clinical diagnostics [74]. Moreover, the molecular imprinting technique has been employed to create synthetic recognition elements that mimic natural biomolecules. These elements are designed to be complementary in shape and functionality to their target analytes, enhancing the specificity of QCM biosensors. This approach has been applied successfully in the detection of various disease-related biomarkers, offering a cost-effective and robust solution for clinical settings [75]. QCM biosensors are particularly advantageous for POC diagnostics due to their ease of use, integration with compact devices, and economic feasibility. These characteristics make them suitable for early disease detection and monitoring, which is critical for managing conditions like SCD [76]. The ongoing development of QCM technology, including the exploration of new bioreceptors and biomarkers, continues to enhance its potential as a diagnostic tool [74]. In summary, while specific studies on QCM for SCD diagnosis were not detailed in the provided abstracts, the general advancements in QCM biosensor technology suggest a promising future for its application in diagnosing and monitoring this condition. The integration of aptamers and molecular imprinting techniques enhances the specificity and sensitivity of QCM biosensors, making them a viable option for clinical diagnostics [74–77].

2.2.10 Genosensors technology

Recent advancements in Genosensors have significantly enhanced the diagnosis of SCD, a genetic disorder characterized by the production of abnormal hemoglobin. Various innovative genosensor technologies have been developed, each offering unique advantages in terms of sensitivity, specificity, and practicality. One promising approach involves the use of aptamer-based electrochemical biosensors. These sensors utilize specific aptamers with high binding affinities for hemoglobin variants HbA and HbS, enabling the differentiation between healthy individuals, SCD patients, and carriers. The aptasensors, which are immobilized on gold electrodes, demonstrate high selectivity and specificity, showing no cross-reactivity with non-specific hemoglobin. This method aligns well with traditional electrophoresis techniques, suggesting its potential for effective SCD diagnosis [78]. Another innovative genosensor employs a colorimetric approach using DNA-CuO nanoparticles to detect SNPs in cell-free fetal DNA. This method is particularly advantageous for prenatal diagnosis, offering a fast, visible, and cost-effective solution with high sensitivity and selectivity for detecting the genetic mutation responsible for SCD [79]. Additionally, a biosensor utilizing CRISPR-Cas9 technology on a graphene field-effect transistor has been developed for the electronic detection of unamplified genomic DNA. This system can rapidly discriminate between wild-type and mutant alleles, providing a quick and efficient method for identifying SCD-related mutations [80]. SPR technology also offers a robust platform for detecting the βS mutation in SCD. This method involves the hybridization of oligonucleotide probes with PCR products, allowing for the precise identification of both homozygous and heterozygous states of the mutation [81]. Lastly, an electrochemical genosensor based on DNA immobilization on gold platforms has been designed for SCD trait determination. This sensor uses electrochemical impedance spectroscopy to distinguish between target and non-target DNA sequences, offering a low-cost and reproducible diagnostic tool [82]. Overall, these genosensor technologies provide diverse and effective strategies for the diagnosis and management of SCD, each contributing to improved early detection and genetic counseling.

2.2.11 The pyrosequencing technique

The pyrosequencing technique has emerged as a valuable tool in the diagnosis and confirmation of SCD, offering a high-throughput, DNA-based approach to detect mutations in the hemoglobin beta (HBB) gene. Unlike traditional approaches such as HPLC, which may falter in differentiating certain hemoglobin variants, recent advancements in pyrosequencing have achieved an impressive 98.7% accuracy in diagnosing HbSS and HbSC genotypes while also effectively identifying heterozygous S variants with a 92.2% accuracy rate. The study underscored the technique's capacity to identify common beta thalassemia mutations prevalent in SCD patients with Sβ-thalassemia [83]. While pyrosequencing offers a robust solution for genetic confirmation of SCD, it is important to consider its integration with other diagnostic methods. For instance, a study on 2,3-diphosphoglycerate (2,3-DPG) detection in SCD patients using mass spectrometry underscores the potential of combining genomic and metabolomic data to enhance disease severity predictions [84]. Additionally, alternative diagnostic approaches, such as the iDAR assay, using a simple, cost-effective, and extraction-free molecular test on buccal swab specimens, provide cost-effective and non-invasive options for SCD screening, particularly in resource-limited settings, though they may not yet match the precision of pyrosequencing in genetic mutation detection [85]. In conclusion, pyrosequencing represents a significant advancement in the genetic diagnosis of SCD, offering high accuracy and the ability to identify complex hemoglobin variants. Its integration with other diagnostic modalities could further enhance its utility in clinical practice, particularly for comprehensive disease management and prognosis.

3. Conclusion

The diagnosis of SCD has been an integral component of clinical laboratory practice for nearly a century. Over recent decades, research endeavors have significantly augmented the understanding of the physiological and biochemical underpinnings of these genetic disorders, thereby enhancing detection methodologies and fostering the development of sophisticated strategies that integrate molecular techniques with traditional biochemical methods. Notwithstanding the methodologies employed, it is imperative that the results are congruent with the clinical presentation. Overall, a majority of hemoglobin variants can be discerned and monitored through red blood cell indices, HPLC results, and IEF. Genetic testing is advocated to corroborate ambiguous cases and to identify atypical and novel variants. Recently, a variety of portable and rapid diagnostic devices have been introduced for the assessment of SCD, encompassing platforms that utilize immune assays, density-based separations, and sensor-based technologies.

Acknowledgements

The author acknowledges the use of typeset.io for the language polishing of the manuscript.

Author details

Mohammed AW. Almorish
Laboratory Hematology and Immunohematology, Department of Hematology, Faculty of Medicine and Health Sciences, Sana'a University, Sana'a, Yemen

*Address all correspondence to: m.almorish@su.edu.ye; almorish70@gmail.com

References

[1] Frömmel C. Newborn screening for sickle cell disease and other hemoglobinopathies: A short review on classical laboratory methods-isoelectric focusing, HPLC, and capillary electrophoresis. International Journal of Neonatal Screening. 2018;**4**(4):39

[2] Kemper AR, Boyle CA, Brosco JP, Grosse SD. Ensuring the life-span benefits of newborn screening. Pediatrics. 2019;**144**(6):e20190904

[3] Laboratories AOPH. Hemoglobinopathies: Current Practices for Screening, Confirmation and Follow up. Atlanta, GA, USA: Centers for Disease Control; 2015 [Accessed: August 7, 2024]

[4] Arishi WA, Alhadrami HA, Zourob M. Techniques for the detection of sickle cell disease a review. Micromachines (Basel). 2021;**12**(5):519

[5] Kavanagh PL, Fasipe TA, Wun T. Sickle cell disease: A review. Journal of the American Medical Association. 2022;**328**(1):57-68. DOI: 10.1001/jama.2022.1023

[6] Piel FB, Hay SI, Gupta S, Weatherall DJ, Williams TN. Global burden of sickle cell anaemia in childreunder five, 2010-2050: Modelling based on demographics, excess mortality, and interventions. PLoS Medicine. 2013;**10**(7):e1001484. DOI: 10.1371/ journal.pmed.1001484

[7] Rouh Aldeen N, Osman AA, Alhabashi MJ, et al. The prevalence of β-thalassemia and other hemoglobinopathies in Kuwaiti premarital screening program: An 11-year experience. Journal of Personalized Medicine. 2021;**11**(10):980. DOI: 10.3390/jpm11100980

[8] Sundd P, Gladwin MT, Novelli EM. Pathophysiology of sickle cell disease. Annual Review of Pathology. 2019;**14**:263-292. DOI: 10.1146/annurevpathmechdis-012418-012838

[9] Gladwin MT, Vichinsky E. Pulmonary complications of sickle cell disease. The New England Journal of Medicine. 2008;**359**(21):2254-2265. DOI: 10.1056/NEJMra0804411

[10] Balde A, Bassene A, Faty L, Soumboundou M, Sall O, Faye Y. Recent artificial intelligence advances in detection and diagnosis of sickle cell disease: A review. In: 2023 IEEE International Conference on Big Data (BigData). Italy: Sorrento; 2023. pp. 3650-3659

[11] Bumgarner R. Overview of dna microarrays: Types, applications, and their future. Current Protocols in Molecular Biology. 2013;**6137**:1-17

[12] Ben Hamda C, Sangeda R, Mwita L, Meintjes A, Nkya S, Panji S, et al. A common molecular signature of patients with sickle cell disease revealed by microarray meta-analysis and a genome-wide association study. PLoS One. 2018;**13**:e0199461

[13] Katsanis SH, Katsanis N. Molecular genetic testing and the future of clinical genomics. Nature Reviews. Genetics. 2013;**14**(6):415-426

[14] Wang X, McKillop WM, Dlugi TA, Faber ML, Alvarez-Argote J, Chambers CB, et al. A mass spectrometry assay for detection of endogenous and lentiviral engineered hemoglobin in cultured cells and sickle cell disease mice. The Journal of Gene Medicine. 2024;**26**(1):e3567

[15] An R, Huang Y, Rocheleau A, Avanaki A, Thota P, Zhang Q, et al.

Multispectral imaging for microChip electrophoresis enables point-of-care newborn hemoglobin variant screening. Heliyon. 2022;**8**(12):e11778

[16] Lukin R, Law JY, Lokhandwala PM. Utility of hemoglobin electrophoresis to distinguish between severe delayed hemolytic transfusion reaction versus hyperhemolysis syndrome. Transfusion and apheresis science : official journal of the World Apheresis Association : official journal of the European Society for Haemapheresis. 2024;**63**(3):103919

[17] Wajcman H. Diagnostic et dépistage de la drépanocystose [diagnosis and screening of sickle cell disease]. La Revue du Praticien. 2004;**54**(14):1543-1547

[18] McGann PT, Hoppe C. The pressing need for point-of-care diagnostics for sickle cell disease: A review of current and future technologies. Blood Cells, Molecules and Diseases. 2017;**67**:104-113

[19] Ou C, Rognerud CL. Diagnosis of hemoglobinopathies: Electrophoresis vs. HPLC. Clinica Chimica Acta. 2001;**313**:187-194

[20] Wajcman H, Moradkhani K. Abnormal haemoglobins: Detection and characterization. The Indian Journal of Medical Research. 2011;**134**:538-546

[21] Nair S. Potential pithfalls in using HPLC and its interpretation in diagnosing HbS. Journal of Rare Diseases Research and Treatment. 2018;**3**:9-12

[22] Clark BE, Thein SL. Molecular diagnosis of haemoglobin disorders. Clinical and Laboratory Haematology. 2004;**26**:159-176

[23] Yue L, Lin M, Chen JT, Zhan XF, Zhong DS, Monte-Nguba SM, et al. Rapid screening for sickle cell disease by polymerase chain reaction-high resolution melting analysis. Molecular Medicine Reports. 2014;**9**:2479-2484

[24] Toye ET, van Marle G, Hutchins W, Abgabiaje O, Okpuzor J. Single tube allele specific PCR: A low cost technique for molecular screening of sickle cell anaemia in Nigeria. African Health Sciences. 2018;**18**:995-1002

[25] Newton CR, Graham A, Heptinstall LE, Powell SJ, Summers C, Kalsheker N, et al. Analysis of any point mutation in DNA. The amplification refractory mutation system (ARMS). Nucleic Acids Research. 1989;**17**:2503-2516

[26] Wu DY, Ugozzoli L, Pal BK, Wallace RB. Allele-specific enzymatic amplification of β-globin genomic DNA for diagnosis of sickle cell anemia. Proceedings of the National Academy of Sciences of the United States of America. 1989;**86**:2757-2760

[27] Wilson JT, Milner PF, Summer ME, Nallaseth FS, Fadel HE, Reindollar RH, et al. Use of restriction endonucleases for mapping the allele for β(s)-globin. Proceedings of the National Academy of Sciences of the United States of America. 1982;**79**:3628-3631

[28] Geever RF, Wilson LB, Nallaseth FS, Milner PF, Bittner M. Direct identification of sickle cell anemia by blot hybridization. Proceedings of the National Academy of Sciences of the United States of America. 1981;**78**:5081-5085

[29] Tripathi GR. A simplified and cheapest method for the diagnosis of sickle cell using whole blood PCR and RFLP in Nepal. Tribhuvan University Journal. 2016;**30**:57-64

[30] Trevino V, Falciani F, Barrera-Saldaña HA. DNA microarrays: A powerful genomic tool for biomedical

and clinical research. Molecular Medicine (Cambridge, Mass.). 2007;**13**(9-10):527-541

[31] Mwesigwa S, Moulds JM, Chen A, Flanagan J, Sheehan VA, George A, et al. Whole-exome sequencing of sickle cell disease patients with hyperhemolysis syndrome suggests a role for rare variation in disease predisposition. Transfusion. 2018;**58**(3):726-735

[32] Suwinski P, Ong C, Ling MHT, Poh YM, Khan AM, Ong HS. Advancing personalized medicine through the application of whole exome sequencing and big data analytics. Frontiers in Genetics. 2019;**10**:49

[33] Rampersaud E, Palmer LE, Hankins JS, Sheehan VA, Bi W, Mulder H, et al. Precision medicine for sickle cell disease through whole genome sequencing. Blood. 2018;**132**:3641

[34] Cardoso V, Moreira R, Mari J, Moreira L. Improving sickle cell disease classification: A fusion of conventional classifiers, segmented images, and convolutional neural networks. In: Proceedings of the 20th National Meeting on Artificial and Computational Intelligence. Porto Alegre: SBC; 2023. pp. 345-358

[35] Goswami NG, Sampathila N, Bairy GM, Goswami A, Siddarama DDB, Belurkar S. Explainable artificial intelligence and deep learning methods for the detection of sickle cell by capturing the digital images of blood smears. Information. 2024;**15**(7):403

[36] Patgiri C, Ganguly A. Machine learning techniques for automatic detection of sickle cell Anemia using adaptive thresholding and contour-based segmentation method. Asian Pacific Journal of Health Sciences. 2022;**9**(4):165-170

[37] Chy TS, Rahaman MA. Automatic sickle cell anemia detection using image processing technique. In: Proceedings of the 2018 IEEE International Conference on Advancement in Electrical and Electronic Engineering (ICAEEE). Gazipur, Bangladesh; 2018. pp. 1-4

[38] Alagu S, Ganesan K, Bhoopathy Bagan K. A novel deep learning approach for sickle cell anemia detection in human RBCs using an improved wrapper-based feature selection technique in microscopic blood smear images. Biomedizinische Technik. Biomedical Engineering. 2022;**68**(2):175-185

[39] Arrojo ML, Lima JMDS, Santos MES, Berbel GM, Murarolli JPZ, Zanelli APRD, et al. Potential clinical application of a flow cytometry method for quantification of fetal hemoglobin (hbf) content in red blood cells (rbcs) in sickle cell disease (scd). Hematology, Transfusion and Cell Therapy. 2023;**45**(4):S74-S75

[40] Butler M, Huq M, Schilke RM, Woolard MD, Stokes KY. A no-lysis flow cytometry protocol to characterize heterotypic aggregates with red blood cells in sickle cell disease. Physiology. 2023;**38**(S1):5734374. DOI: 10.1152/physiol.2023.38.s1.5734374

[41] An R, Gurkan UA. Emerging functional microfluidic assays for the study of thromboinflammation in sickle cell disease. Current Opinion in Hematology. 2022;**29**(6):327-334

[42] Özpolat T, Chang TC, Wu X, St. John AE, Konkle BA, Chen J, et al. Phenotypic analysis of erythrocytes in sickle cell disease using imaging flow cytometry. Cytometry. Part A: The Journal of the International Society for Analytical Cytology. 2022;**101**(5):448-457

[43] Davis BH. Assay for "fetal hemoglobin levels" in erythrocytes:

Impact of new in vitro diagnostics regulation and expanded applications in sickle cell disease management. American Journal of Hematology. 2020;**95**(11):1230-1232

[44] Fertrin KY, Samsel L, van Beers EJ, Mendelsohn L, Kato GJ, McCoy JP. Sickle cell imaging flow cytometry assay (SIFCA). Imaging Flow Cytometry. 2016;**1389**:279-292

[45] Cai C, Nedosekin DA, Menyaev YA, Sarimollaoglu M, Proskurnin MA, Zharov VP. Photoacoustic flow cytometry for single sickle cell detection In vitro and In vivo. Analytical Cellular Pathology. 2016;**2016**:2642361

[46] Liua J, Qianga Y, Alvarezb O, Dua E. Electrical impedance microflow cytometry with oxygen control for detection of sickle cells. Sensors and Actuators B: Chemical. 2018;**255**:2392-2398

[47] Dadelahi A, Jackson T, Agarwal AM, Lin L, Rets AV, Ng DP. Applications of flow cytometry in diagnosis and evaluation of red blood cell disorders. Clinics in Laboratory Medicine. 2024;**44**(3):495-509

[48] Patwardhan AA, Oshabaheebwa S, Delianides CA, Sekyonda Z, Patel AP, Evans EN, et al. Comparison of devices that measure sickle red cell deformability. Blood. 2023;**142**(Suppl. 1):3669

[49] Chaturvedi P, Shah SR. Mathematical analysis for the flow of sickle red blood cells in microvessels for bio medical application. The Yale Journal of Biology and Medicine. 2023;**96**(1):13-21

[50] Chaturvedi P, Kumar R, Shah SR. Bio-mechanical and bio-rheological aspects of sickle red cells in microcirculation: A mathematical modelling approach. Fluids. 2021;**6**(9):322

[51] Williams DC, Wood DK. High-throughput quantification of red blood cell deformability and oxygen saturation to probe mechanisms of sickle cell disease. Proceedings of the National Academy of Sciences of the United States of America. 2023;**120**(48):e2313755120

[52] Chang MM, Natoli ME, Wilkinson AF, Tubman VN, Airewele GE, Richards-Kortum RR. A multiplexed, allele-specific recombinase polymerase amplification assay with lateral flow readout for sickle cell disease detection. Lab on a Chip. 2024;**24**(17):4115-4127. DOI: 10.1039/d4lc00281d

[53] Kim J, Shin MS, Shin J, Kim HM, Pham XH, Park SM, et al. Recent trends in lateral flow immunoassays with optical nanoparticles. International Journal of Molecular Sciences. 2023;**24**(11):9600

[54] Lancia M, Pang T, Crawford A, Wing J, Mehta K, Cheng X. A novel E-junction lateral flow immunoassay for widespread sickle cell screening in low and middle-income countries. In: Proceedings of the 2020 IEEE Global Humanitarian Technology Conference (GHTC). Seattle, WA, USA; 2020. pp. 1-7

[55] McGann PT, Schaefer BA, Paniagua M, Howard TA, Ware RE. Characteristics of a rapid, point-of-care lateral flow immunoassay for the diagnosis of sickle cell disease. American Journal of Hematology. 2016;**91**(2):205-210

[56] Okeke CO, Chianumba RI, Isa H, Asala S, Nnodu OE. Using dried blood spot on HemoTypeSC™, a new frontier for newborn screening for sickle cell disease in Nigeria. Frontiers in Genetics. 2022;**13**:1013858

[57] Kasai ET, Kadima JN, Alworong'a Opara JP, Boemer F, Dresse MF,

Makani J, et al. Pairing parents and offspring's HemoTypeSC test to validate results and confirm sickle cell pedigree: A case study in Kisangani, the Democratic Republic of the Congo. Hematology. 2022;**27**(1):853-859

[58] Goreke U, Bode A, Yaman S, Gurkan UA, Durmus NG. Size and density measurements of single sickle red blood cells using microfluidic magnetic levitation. Lab on a Chip. 2022;**22**(4):683-696

[59] Kumar AA, Patton MR, Hennek JW, Lee SYR, D'alesio-Spina G, Yang X, et al. Density-based separation in multiphase systems provides a simple method to identify sickle cell disease. Proceedings of the National Academy of Sciences of the United States of America. 2014;**111**:14864-14869

[60] Alapan Y, Fraiwan A, Kucukal E, Hasan MN, Ung R, Kim M, et al. Emerging point-of-care technologies for sickle cell disease screening and monitoring. Expert Review of Medical Devices. 2016;**13**:1073-1093

[61] Kumar AA, Chunda-Liyoka C, Hennek JW, Mantina H, Lee SYR, Patton MR, et al. Evaluation of a density-based rapid diagnostic test for sickle cell disease in a clinical setting in Zambia. PLoS One. 2014;**9**(12):e114540

[62] Mendez SR, Marti WB, Ershler AS, Zik C. How sensitive is the sickle prep? Clinical implications. Blood. 2023;**142**(Suppl. 1):5335

[63] Kumar R, Mishra S, Gwal A, Shanmugam R. Evaluation of paper-based point of care screening test for sickle cell disease. Indian Journal of Clinical Biochemistry: IJCB. 2022;**37**(2):185-191

[64] Hasan MN, Fraiwan A, An R, Alapan Y, Ung R, Akkus A, et al. Paper-based microchip electrophoresis for point-of-care hemoglobin testing. The Analyst. 2020;**145**(7):2525-2542

[65] Yassen K, Omer N, Alsahaf F, Al Amer F, Alhamad F, Alherz I, et al. Comparing non-invasive spectrophotometry to hematology analysis for Hemoglobin measurements in sickle cell disease patients. Journal of Clinical Medicine. 2023;**12**(24):7517

[66] Srivastava S, Radhika NK, Srinivasan R, Nambison NK, Gorthi SS. Diagnosis of Sickle Cell Anemia Using AutoML on UV-Vis Absorbance Spectroscopy Data. 2021;**arXiv**:2111.12711

[67] Dai H, Yin C, Ye X, Jiang B, Ran M, Cao Z, et al. A possible pathogenetic factor of sickle-cell disease based on fluorescent analysis via an optofluidic resonator. Scientific Reports. 2017;**7**(1):3174

[68] Park SM, Ji Y, Kwon S, Leem JW, O'Brien ARW, Wang Y, et al. Remote blood hemoglobin monitoring with hyperspectral color truthing for advancing sickle cell care. Blood. 2023;**142**(Suppl. 1):2277

[69] Mostashari G, Quang T, Parker HE, Hill M, Parekh D, Keel A, et al. Exploring near infrared spectroscopy as a tool for monitoring tissue hemodynamics for patients with sickle cell disease. Blood. 2023;**142**(Suppl. 1):3862

[70] Tieying X, Lizarralde-Iragorri MA, Charlot B, Roman J, Français O, El Nemer W, et al. Bioimpedance single cell sensing of low and high density sickle erythrocytes using microfluidics. Biosensors and Bioelectronics: X. 2022;**10**:100140

[71] Ertuğrul Uygun HD. Impedimetric CRISPR-dCas9 based biosensor system

for sickle cell anemia mutation. JOTCSA. 2022;**9**(3):631-638

[72] Qiang Y, Liu J, Dieujuste D, Du E. Electrical impedance detection of sickle cell vaso-occlusion in microfluidic capillary structures. bioRxiv. 2020;**07**:227215. DOI: 10.1101/2020.07.29.227215

[73] Liu J, Qiang Y, Du E. Dielectric spectroscopy of red blood cells in sickle cell disease. Electrophoresis. 2021;**42**(5):667-675

[74] Vashist SK, Luong JHT. Chapter 13—Quartz crystal microbalance–based sensors. In: Vashist SK, Luong JHT, editors. Handbook of Immunoassay Technologies. Cambridge, US: Academic Press; 2018. pp. 333-357

[75] Akgönüllü S, Özgür E, Denizli A. Quartz crystal microbalance-based aptasensors for medical diagnosis. Micromachines. 2022;**13**(9):1441

[76] Akgönüllü S, Özgür E, Denizli A. Recent advances in quartz crystal microbalance biosensors based on the molecular imprinting technique for disease-related biomarkers. Chemsensors. 2022;**10**(3):106

[77] Prakrankamanant P. Quartz crystal microbalance biosensors: Prospects for point-of-care diagnostics. Journal of the Medical Association of Thailand = Chotmaihet Thangphaet. 2014;**97**(Suppl. 4):S56-S64

[78] Arishi WA, Eissa S, Al-Kattan K, Zourob M. Aptamer-based label-free electrochemical biosensors for the diagnosis of sickle cell anemia. Biosensors and Bioelectronics: X. 2023;**14**:100389

[79] Kasiri M, Rahaie M. A visible and colorimetric nanobiosensor based on DNA-CuO nanoparticle for detection of single nucleotide polymorphism involved in sickle cell anemia disease. Materials Today Communications. 2021;**27**:102423

[80] Balderston S, Taulbee JJ, Celaya E, et al. Discrimination of single-point mutations in unamplified genomic DNA via Cas9 immobilized on a graphene field-effect transistor. Nature Biomedical Engineering. 2021;**5**:713-725

[81] Breveglieri G, D'Aversa E, Cosenza LC, Boutou E, Balassopoulou A, Voskaridou E, et al. Detection of the sickle hemoglobin allele using a surface plasmon resonance based biosensor. Sensors and Actuators. B Chemical. 2019;**296**:126604

[82] Brazaca LC, Bramorski CB, Cancino-Bernardi J, Janegitz BC. A genosensor for sickle cell Anemia trait determination. Electroanalysis. 2017;**29**:773-777

[83] De Martino CC, Alencar CS, Loureiro P, Carneiro-Proietti ABF, Máximo CA, Mota RA, et al. Use of an automated pyrosequencing technique for confirmation of sickle cell disease. PLoS One. 2019;**14**(12):e0216020

[84] Van Der Veen S, Van Dijk M, Jans J, Verhoeven-Duif N, et al. P-023: 2,3-diphosphoglycerate detection via direct infusion high resolution mass spectrometry correlates with quantitative detection in blood of patients with sickle cell disease. Hema. 2022;**6**(Suppl.):28-29

[85] Thakur P, Gupta P, Bhargava N, Soni R, Varma Gottumukkala N, Goswami SG, et al. A simple, cost-effective, and extraction-free molecular diagnostic test for sickle cell disease using a noninvasive buccal swab specimen for a limited-resource setting. Diagnostics (Basel, Switzerland). 2022;**12**(7):1765

Chapter 3

Perspective Chapter: Recent Developments in the Treatment of Sickle Cell Disease

Mohammed Abdulwahid Almorish and Ali A. Alyahawi

Abstract

Recent developments in the treatment of sickle cell disease (SCD) have been marked by significant advancements in gene therapy and pharmacotherapy, offering new hope for patients suffering from this debilitating condition. Therapeutic interventions that modify disease, including hydroxyurea, L-glutamine, voxelotor, and crizanlizumab, have been shown to diminish the frequency of pain crises and mitigate severe complications. Presently, allogeneic hematopoietic stem cell transplantation (HSCT) utilizing matched sibling donors represents the sole standard curative approach; nevertheless, a limited percentage of patients possess such compatible donors. The food and drug administration (FDA) approval of novel gene editing therapies and the introduction of new pharmacological agents have transformed the therapeutic landscape, providing both curative and disease-modifying options. These innovations, however, come with challenges related to accessibility and cost, which need to be addressed to ensure equitable treatment distribution.

Keywords: sickle cell disease (SCD), gene editing, crizanlizumab, voxelotor, L-glutamine

1. Introduction

SCD results from a singular nucleotide substitution in the beta-globin gene, leading to the incorporation of valine at the sixth position of the amino acid sequence as opposed to the typical glutamic acid, thus producing hemoglobin S (HbS) [1]. In conditions of low oxygen saturation, HbS undergoes polymerization, resulting in the distortion of erythrocytes into a sickle morphology [2]. These erythrocytes containing HbS exhibit a diminished capacity for oxygen transport. The morphological alteration of the erythrocytes, along with an augmented expression of surface adhesion molecules, may precipitate vascular occlusion, painful vaso-occlusive crises (VOC), and protracted damage to various tissues and organs [3].

SCD ranks among the most common inherited monogenic disorders on a global scale. Its prevalence is notably higher among Black Americans relative to other ethnic groups. Estimates suggest that over 20 million individuals are affected worldwide, with approximately 80,000 to 100,000 cases in the United States alone, where around 3000 children are born with the condition each year [4].

Advancements in treatment have improved life expectancy; however, individuals with SCD still exhibit a markedly lower life expectancy of 54 years compared to 76 years in controls [5]. Hydroxyurea, the sole FDA-approved therapy for SCD since 1998, enhances hemoglobin F levels, thereby mitigating deoxygenation and polymerization of red blood cells (RBCs), although adherence rates remain suboptimal [6]. Recently, three novel medications—L-glutamine, crizanlizumab, and voxelotor—have been authorized, each demonstrating efficacy in reducing pain crises and improving clinical outcomes in SCD patients. Recent curative research emphasizes gene therapy as a corrective measure for genetic disorders, with this chapter reviewing both traditional SCD treatments and innovative future options that inspire optimism for SCD patients [7].

2. Recent developments in treatments of SCD

2.1 Hemoglobin F induction therapies

2.1.1 Hydroxyurea

Recent developments in the use of hydroxyurea for treating patients with SCD highlight its potential benefits and challenges. Hydroxyurea is primarily recognized for its ability to increase HbF levels, which can ameliorate the symptoms and complications associated with SCD by reducing the aggregation of HbS [8].

A randomized phase II trial, Hydroxyurea Prevent, demonstrated that Hydroxyurea might significantly reduce the incidence of central nervous system injuries in young children with SCD, suggesting a profound neuroprotective effect and supporting further phase III studies [9]. However, the response to Hydroxyurea is not uniform across all patients. Up to 30% of patients may not respond effectively, with genetic factors playing a crucial role in this variability. Research has identified several genetic loci, such as CYP2C9, CYP2E1, and BCL11A, that influence Hydroxyurea response, indicating the potential for personalized medicine approaches to optimize treatment [10]. Additionally, while Hydroxyurea is generally safe, its impact on fertility, particularly ovarian reserve, has been a concern. A study examining ovarian follicle density found no significant reduction in ovarian reserve among girls and young women with SCD treated with hydroxyurea, suggesting that fertility preservation measures may not be necessary before treatment initiation [11]. Despite its benefits, hydroxyurea uptake remains low. A pharmacist-managed protocol significantly improved hydroxyurea uptake and optimization among SCD patients, increasing the proportion of patients reaching the maximum tolerated dose and enhancing HbF levels [12]. This approach underscores the importance of structured support systems in improving treatment outcomes.

Hydroxyurea continues to be a cornerstone in SCD management, with ongoing research focusing on optimizing its use through genetic insights and supportive care protocols. While promising, further studies are needed to fully understand its mechanisms, particularly concerning DNA methylation and long-term effects [8].

2.1.2 Decitabine

Recent advancements in decitabine administration for SCD emphasize improving its bioavailability and therapeutic outcomes via novel formulations. SCD involves the polymerization of HbS, resulting in the deformation of RBCs. HbF can disrupt this polymerization; however, it is generally repressed in adults by DNA methyltransferase 1 (DNMT1) [13, 14].

Decitabine, a DNMT1 inhibitor, enhances HbF levels in SCD patients. Its efficacy is constrained by rapid catabolism by cytidine deaminase (CDA). Tetrahydrouridine (THU) inhibits CDA, increasing decitabine's bioavailability. Recent investigations have assessed oral formulations of decitabine and THU, showing favorable pharmacokinetics and pharmacodynamics for DNMT1-targeted therapy. These formulations are well tolerated, with no significant adverse effects reported, and are undergoing phase 2 evaluations [13, 14]. A phase 1 clinical trial assessed the safety and efficacy of oral THU-decitabine in SCD patients. The findings indicated that the combination was safe, effectively enhancing HbF levels, thereby improving erythropoiesis and decreasing hemolysis and inflammation markers. The trial reported no significant non-hematologic toxicity, with the treatment correlating with enhanced RBC quality and increased total hemoglobin levels [14]. While promising, further research is required to evaluate the clinical efficacy and risks of this treatment. The emergence of decitabine as a non-cytotoxic epigenetic therapy marks a notable progression in SCD management, enhancing current treatments and possibly benefiting patient outcomes [7].

2.1.3 HDAC inhibitors

Recent studies on histone deacetylase (HDAC) inhibitors for SCD treatment reveal their potential in inducing HbF, a therapeutic avenue that mitigates SCD symptoms by reducing red blood cell sickling. Specifically, the selective HDAC1 and HDAC2 inhibitor ACY-957 has been shown to enhance γ-globin mRNA and HbF levels through GATA2 gene activation, underscoring the significance of histone acetylation in this process [15]. Subsequent research has validated that the suppression of HDAC1 or HDAC2 can enhance γ-globin expression without impacting cell proliferation or the cell cycle, positioning these inhibitors as promising candidates for combinatorial therapies [16]. The synergistic effect observed when HDAC inhibitors are paired with hydroxyurea suggests an increased therapeutic potential for SCD treatment, necessitating further clinical exploration to ascertain the safety and efficacy of these agents alongside existing treatments [17].

2.1.4 Benserazide

Recent developments in the use of benserazide for treating patients with SCD have shown promising potential, although further research is needed to establish its efficacy. Benserazide, traditionally used in Parkinson's disease, has been identified as a potential inducer of HbF, which can ameliorate the clinical severity of β-hemoglobinopathies, including SCD [18, 19]. In preclinical studies, benserazide has demonstrated the ability to activate fetal globin gene expression, leading to increased HbF production in erythroid progenitors from hemoglobinopathy patients, transgenic mice, and anemic baboons [19].

These findings suggest that benserazide could be a viable therapeutic candidate for SCD, as increased HbF levels can reduce the sickling of red blood cells and associated complications. However, an observational study involving patients on benserazide for Parkinson's disease did not show a significant increase in HbF or F-cell percentages, indicating that the drug's efficacy in inducing HbF in humans remains uncertain [19]. Despite this, the study confirmed the long-term safety and tolerability of benserazide, even at high doses, supporting its potential for further clinical trials in SCD patients [18]. Currently, the BENeFiTS trial (NCT04432623) is underway to assess the efficacy of benserazide in beta-thalassemia and SCD patients, initiated in 2020 and projected to conclude by December 2024, focusing on various dosages and evaluating treatment-related adverse events, plasma concentrations, and hematological parameters such as HbF levels [20]. Benserazide demonstrates promise in treating SCD by stimulating HbF production, its therapeutic efficacy necessitates further validation through clinical trials, bolstered by its proven safety and preclinical achievements.

2.2 Anti-HbS polymerization therapies

2.2.1 Voxelotor

Voxelotor (GBT440), a first-in-class HbS polymerization inhibitor, has shown promising developments in the treatment of SCD. Recent studies highlight its efficacy in increasing hemoglobin levels and reducing hemolysis, which are critical in managing SCD symptoms such as chronic anemia and vaso-occlusive crises [VOCs] [21, 22].

The PROSPECT study, a real-world registry, reported that voxelotor treatment led to a mean increase in hemoglobin levels by 1.5 g/dL and reductions in hemolytic markers, such as reticulocyte count and bilirubin levels, in a cohort of 150 patients [21]. These findings align with the HOPE and HOPE-KIDS 1 trials, confirming voxelotor's effectiveness and safety in a broader patient population [22]. Additionally, voxelotor's mechanism of action, which improves red blood cell deformability, enhances microcirculatory flow and reduces the risk of VOCs, as demonstrated through mathematical modeling and microfluidics-based diagnostics [23]. Long-term safety and efficacy data from the HOPE open-label extension study further support voxelotor's role in SCD management. Over 168 weeks, patients maintained improved hemoglobin levels and stable hemolytic markers, with no new safety concerns identified [24]. However, a study on thromboembolic events raised concerns about potential risks associated with increased hemoglobin levels, noting a 12% incidence of such events in patients on voxelotor, particularly in those with a history of venous thromboembolism [24].

In pediatric patients, voxelotor has been shown to reduce cerebral hemodynamic impairments, suggesting potential benefits beyond hematological improvements [25]. Despite these positive outcomes, the risk of thromboembolic events necessitates further investigation to fully understand voxelotor's safety profile and optimize its use in SCD treatment [24]. Overall, voxelotor represents a significant advancement in SCD therapy, offering improved clinical outcomes with a generally favorable safety profile, though continued monitoring and research are essential.

2.2.2 GBT021601

GBT021601 is a next-generation HbS polymerization inhibitor currently under investigation for the treatment of SCD. This compound is designed to improve hemoglobin [Hb]-oxygen affinity and stabilize Hb in its oxygenated state, thereby inhibiting polymerization and potentially reducing treatment burden compared to existing therapies like voxelotor [26, 27]. Recent preliminary results from a multicenter phase 2/3 study indicate that GBT021601 is well tolerated and effective in increasing hemoglobin levels in patients with SCD. In a 12-week dose-finding study [Part A], patients receiving 100 mg and 150 mg doses of GBT021601 showed mean increases in Hb of 2.67 g/dL and 3.17 g/dL, respectively. These improvements were accompanied by favorable trends in hemolysis markers and a reduction in adherent cells, which may correlate with a decreased risk of VOCs [26, 27]. Pharmacodynamic data further support these findings, showing improvements in RBC parameters such as hematocrit and RBC deformability, with near normalization of these parameters over the 12-week period [27]. Additionally, preclinical studies in murine models have demonstrated that GBT021601 reduces RBC sickling, improves RBC deformability, and prolongs RBC half-life, suggesting its potential to improve overall RBC health and oxygen delivery [28, 29]. While these results are promising, it is important to note that the study is ongoing, and long-term effects and safety profiles are yet to be fully established. The current data support the continued clinical development of GBT021601 as a potential treatment for SCD, with the potential to offer a more effective and less burdensome therapeutic option compared to existing treatments [26–28]. Further research will be necessary to confirm these findings and to explore the long-term benefits and risks associated with GBT021601 therapy.

2.3 Pyruvate kinase activators

2.3.1 Mitapivat

Mitapivat [AG-348] is an oral, allosteric activator of pyruvate kinase (PK), which plays a crucial role in RBC metabolism by increasing adenosine triphosphate [ATP] levels and decreasing 2,3-DPG levels. These changes enhance hemoglobin's oxygen affinity and reduce sickling in SCD patients [30, 31].

Clinical studies have shown that mitapivat significantly impacts the metabolome, lipidome, and proteome of RBCs in SCD patients. It improves hematologic parameters and sickling kinetics, with sustained increases in hemoglobin levels and reductions in hemolysis markers over extended treatment periods [31, 32]. In a phase 2 study, mitapivat altered a broad spectrum of metabolites, indicating its potential to modify disease pathways beyond glycolysis [30]. Long-term safety and efficacy data from an extension of a phase 1 study revealed that mitapivat is generally well-tolerated, with no treatment-emergent adverse events leading to discontinuation. The most common adverse events were VOCs, which were consistent with known triggers rather than the drug itself [32]. The study also reported sustained improvements in hemoglobin levels and RBC deformability, suggesting a durable therapeutic effect [32]. Moreover, the RISE UP phase 2/3 trial emphasizes a patient-centric approach, integrating patient feedback into the trial design to enhance participation and address patient needs, such as pain management and fatigue [33].

This approach may improve trial outcomes and patient engagement, highlighting the importance of involving patients in clinical research. Overall, mitapivat represents a novel, disease-modifying therapy for SCD, with evidence supporting its efficacy in improving RBC function and reducing sickling. However, further studies are needed to confirm these findings and optimize treatment protocols [30–33].

2.3.2 Etavopivat

Etavopivat [FT-4202], an investigational oral selective erythrocyte PK activator, is being developed for the treatment of SCD. Recent studies have demonstrated its potential to improve RBC health and reduce complications associated with SCD. In a multicenter, phase 1 study, etavopivat was administered to patients with SCD at a dose of 400 mg once daily for 12 weeks. The treatment resulted in significant increases in hemoglobin levels, with a mean maximal increase of 1.6 g/dL, and improved RBC physiology, including increased ATP levels and decreased 2,3-DPG levels, which are associated with reduced hemolysis and improved RBC lifespan [34, 35].

The safety profile of etavopivat was generally favorable, with most adverse events being mild to moderate and consistent with the underlying SCD. Serious adverse events were reported in a few patients, but these were not directly related to the treatment [34, 35]. The ongoing HIBISCUS-KIDS study aims to evaluate the pharmacokinetics and safety of etavopivat in pediatric patients, with a focus on reducing VOCs and improving overall RBC health [36]. Etavopivat's mechanism of action involves enhancing PK activity, which decreases 2,3-DPG and increases ATP, thereby improving hemoglobin-oxygen affinity and reducing sickling of RBCs. This mechanism has been validated in both nonhuman primates and human subjects, showing promise in reducing vaso-occlusion and improving anemia in SCD patients [37]. Overall, etavopivat has shown potential as a novel therapeutic option for SCD, with evidence supporting its ability to improve RBC health and reduce disease complications. Further studies, including the ongoing phase 2/3 Hibiscus trial, are necessary to confirm these findings and establish its long-term efficacy and safety in both adult and pediatric populations [37, 38].

2.4 Anti-adhesion therapies

2.4.1 Crizanlizumab

Crizanlizumab-tmca (ADAKVEO), a humanized monoclonal antibody targeting P-selectin, has been explored for its potential to reduce VOCs in patients with SCD. Despite initial promise, recent developments have highlighted mixed results regarding its efficacy and safety. The European Medicines Agency revoked the marketing authorization for crizanlizumab due to the STAND study's failure to show significant differences in VOC rates compared to placebo [39]. This study, a large Phase III trial, found no statistically significant reduction in VOCs with crizanlizumab at doses of 5 mg/kg or 7.5 mg/kg compared to placebo, although it did confirm the drug's activity on P-selectin levels [40]. Similarly, a German retrospective analysis reported an increase in VOCs over time in patients treated with crizanlizumab, alongside a high incidence of serious adverse events, further supporting the revocation decision [39]. Conversely, other studies have reported more favorable outcomes. The SOLACE-adults study demonstrated a reduction in VOC rates from baseline with long-term crizanlizumab treatment, suggesting potential sustained efficacy [41]. Additionally, a real-world study indicated improvements in patient-reported outcomes and a reduction in opioid use, although no significant changes in laboratory parameters were observed [42]. A case report also highlighted crizanlizumab's potential in managing priapism, a complication of SCD, though it noted the risk of infusion-related VOCs [43].

Overall, while crizanlizumab shows some promise in specific contexts, its efficacy in reducing VOCs remains inconsistent across studies. The discrepancies may stem from differences in study design, patient populations, and healthcare settings. The safety profile is generally consistent with known adverse events, but serious events and economic considerations pose challenges. Further research is needed to clarify its role in SCD management, particularly in light of the contrasting findings from different studies [39–43].

2.4.2 Epeleuton

Epeleuton, a synthetic ω-3 fatty acid, has shown promise in preclinical studies by modulating inflammatory responses and reducing hemolysis and sickling in SCD models. It achieves this by reprogramming the lipidomic pattern of target organs toward a pro-resolving state, thereby protecting against systemic and local inflammation and improving RBC characteristics [44]. A Phase 2 open-label study is currently underway to evaluate the pharmacokinetics, pharmacodynamics, and safety of epeleuton in SCD patients. This study involves administering epeleuton to patients with confirmed SCD diagnoses and aims to assess changes in hemoglobin levels, hemolytic markers, and rates of VOCs over a 16-week treatment period [45]. The study's design allows for the concomitant use of hydroxyurea, a standard SCD treatment, which may provide insights into epeleuton's additive or synergistic effects. Epeleuton's mechanism of action includes reducing endothelial adhesion of RBCs, a critical factor in VOCs, as demonstrated in microfluidic studies using SCD patient samples. These studies showed that epeleuton significantly decreased RBC adhesion to heme-activated endothelium, suggesting its potential to mitigate one of the primary causes of VOCs in SCD [46]. Epeleuton, with its favorable safety profile and oral administration, presents a more accessible alternative that could complement existing treatments and address multiple aspects of SCD pathology [20].

Epeleuton represents a promising development in SCD treatment, with ongoing clinical trials expected to further elucidate its efficacy and safety profile. Its ability to target inflammation and RBC adhesion could provide significant benefits to SCD patients, potentially reducing the frequency and severity of VOCs and improving overall disease management.

2.4.3 Famotidine

Recent advancements in famotidine, a histamine type 2 [H2] receptor antagonist for SCD treatment, indicate a reduction in plasma soluble P-selectin levels. Allali et al. found that famotidine significantly decreased median plasma P-selectin in SCD children over 29 days. This reduction implies a potential role for famotidine in minimizing vaso-occlusive incidents, though no impacts on other adhesion molecules or inflammatory markers, aside from reduced reticulocyte count, were noted. Notably, famotidine was reported to be safe, with no adverse events documented. Nonetheless, the authors stress the necessity for randomized controlled trials to evaluate famotidine's efficacy in preventing vaso-occlusion in SCD patients [47]. While famotidine shows potential, it is not yet a standard treatment for SCD. The investigation of famotidine is part of broader efforts to create more effective and accessible therapies [20].

2.4.4 Inclacumab

Inclacumab, a fully human monoclonal antibody targeting P-selectin, is under investigation for its potential to treat SCD by reducing VOCs, a major complication of the disease. The THRIVE studies are global, multicenter, phase 3 trials designed to assess inclacumab's efficacy and safety in SCD patients. They investigate the antibody's role in inhibiting sickle RBCs, platelets, and leukocyte adhesion to the endothelium to potentially decrease VOC incidence [48, 49]. The THRIVE-131 trial enrolls roughly 240 participants receiving intravenous inclacumab or placebo biweekly for 48 weeks, focusing on VOC rates as the primary endpoint. Conversely, the THRIVE-132 trial includes approximately 280 participants receiving a single inclacumab or placebo dose post-VOC, with readmission rates for VOCs within 90 days as the primary endpoint. Additionally, an open-label extension study THRIVE-133 is conducted to evaluate inclacumab's long-term safety [49]. In vitro studies indicate that inclacumab markedly inhibits cell adhesion to P-selectin in a dose-dependent manner. This implies that inclacumab may significantly hinder sickle cell adhesion to the endothelium, potentially averting VOCs [50]. However, ongoing studies necessitate caution as final outcomes remain unpublished. Preliminary findings propose inclacumab as a potentially beneficial therapeutic for SCD in reducing VOCs, yet additional research is essential to verify its long-term efficacy and safety [48–50].

2.5 Intravenous gamma globulin [IVIG]

Recent studies on intravenous gamma globulin [IVIG] in the treatment of SCD demonstrate notable efficacy, particularly in managing pain crises, as a Phase I trial revealed that IVIG doses ranging from 200 to 800 mg/kg substantially diminished Mac-1 functionality on neutrophils in sickle cell anemia [SCA] patients, with the most significant effects observed at lower doses [200–400 mg/kg] [51]. This implies that IVIG may diminish neutrophil-red blood cell interactions, which are crucial in vaso-occlusive pathophysiology of SCD. The research also revealed that higher IVIG doses [600–800 mg/kg] could cause adverse effects, while lower doses did not appreciably elevate neutrophil and leukocyte counts, suggesting targeted inhibition of Mac-1 rather than overall neutrophil suppression [51, 52]. IVIG constitutes a valuable adjunctive intervention for alleviating acute pain episodes in SCD, necessitating further investigation to refine dosage and mitigate side effects while synergizing with other novel therapies focused on symptomatic relief and potential curative strategies for SCD.

2.6 Gene therapy

Gene therapy is being studied as a treatment for SCD. Advances in genomic sequencing have facilitated the understanding of Hb regulation, and genome modification of hematopoietic stem cells presents potential alternative therapies for SCD. CD34+ serves as a marker for identifying hematopoietic and progenitor stem cells in bone marrow transplant research to create targeted genetic therapies [53]. Gene editing methods employing gene transfer vectors have been refined to enhance the expression of normal or anti-sickling globins for SCD treatment. Genome association studies indicate that the BCL11A gene influences HbF production, with its downregulation leading to increased HbF levels [54]. Gene therapy has demonstrated a reduction in the incidence of SCD-related complications such as VOCs, acute chest syndrome, and graft versus host disease (GVHD) from HSCT [55].

2.6.1 BCH-BB694

The development of BCH-BB694, a lentiviral vector targeting BCL11A to enhance gamma-globin gene expression, marks notable progress in gene therapy for SCD by increasing fetal hemoglobin production to counteract the effects of defective adult hemoglobin [54].

Preclinical investigations reveal that BCH-BB694 significantly enhances HbF levels through high vector copy numbers and gene marking without compromising the growth, differentiation, or engraftment of modified cells, while exhibiting no genotoxicity, thereby affirming its safety and efficacy in the context of evolving gene therapy approaches for SCD, including CRISPR-Cas and base editing techniques aimed at γ-globin reactivation and HBB gene mutation correction [7, 55]. These approaches are essential due to the limitations of existing therapies, including the lack of suitable sibling donors for hematopoietic stem cell transplants and the substantial costs of novel gene therapies [56]. Although BCH-BB694 exhibits potential, it remains in the preclinical stage, necessitating further clinical trials to validate its safety and effectiveness in human subjects. The continuous research and development of these therapies highlight the necessity for interdisciplinary collaboration to enhance treatment approaches for SCD patients. As these therapies advance, they promise to offer more accessible and effective solutions for individuals afflicted with SCD [7, 57].

2.6.2 Casgevy/Exa-Cel [CTX001]

Recent developments in the treatment of SCD have seen the introduction of Casgevy/Exa-Cel [CTX001], a CRISPR/Cas9-based gene therapy that offers a potentially curative approach for patients aged 12 years and older with recurrent VOCs [58]. This therapy involves ex vivo gene editing of autologous CD34+ hematopoietic stem and progenitor cells (HSPCs) to reactivate HbF synthesis by targeting the erythroid-specific enhancer region of BCL11A, a transcription factor that represses γ-globin expression postnatally [59]. Clinical trials have demonstrated significant efficacy, with 97% of patients achieving freedom from severe VOCs for at least 12 consecutive months, and 100% avoiding hospitalizations for VOCs over the same period. The therapy has shown a favorable safety profile, consistent with the effects of myeloablative conditioning and autologous HSPC transplantation, with no reported cases of cancer or serious adverse events directly related to the gene editing process [58, 59].

The FDA's approval of Casgevy marks a significant milestone as the first CRISPR/Cas9 gene therapy for SCD, highlighting its transformative potential in SCD management by reducing the need for recurrent transfusions and transplants, thus improving patients' quality of life [60, 61]. However, ethical considerations and regulatory challenges remain, particularly concerning equitable access and the long-term implications of CRISPR technology [60, 62]. Despite the high upfront costs associated with Casgevy, innovative payment models are being explored to address financial barriers and ensure broader access to this groundbreaking therapy. Overall, Casgevy/Exa-Cel represents a promising advancement in the treatment of SCD, offering hope for a functional cure and setting a precedent for future applications of gene editing in medicine [59, 60, 62].

2.6.3 Lyfgenia/Lov-Cel [BB305]

Recent advancements in the treatment of SCD have been marked by the emergence of gene therapies like Lyfgenia, or lovotibeglogene autotemcel (lovo-cel). This therapy, approved by the FDA in December 2023, is designed for patients aged 12 and older who experience recurrent vaso-occlusive events (VOEs) [63, 64].

Lovo-cel utilizes a lentiviral vector to transduce autologous hematopoietic stem cells with a modified β-globin gene, which produces an anti-sickling hemoglobin, HbA T87Q, offering a potentially curative approach to SCD [63, 65]. Clinical trials, particularly the phase 1/2 HGB-206 and phase 3 HGB-210 studies, have demonstrated the efficacy and safety of lovo-cel. These trials reported a significant reduction in VOEs, with 90.9% of patients achieving complete resolution of VOEs within 6–18 months post-infusion [65]. Additionally, patients experienced improvements in hemoglobin levels and health-related quality of life, with reductions in pain intensity and fatigue [65].

From an economic perspective, lovo-cel has been shown to extend life expectancy by an average of 23.84 years compared to standard care, with substantial quality-adjusted life-year gains. However, the high cost of treatment, approximately $3.28 million per patient, poses challenges for widespread adoption, despite its cost-effectiveness from a societal perspective [66]. While lovo-cel represents a significant advancement in SCD treatment, challenges remain regarding access and equity, particularly in regions like Africa where SCD prevalence is high. Ensuring that these therapies reach those in need requires addressing logistical and political barriers [64]. Moreover, ongoing research is necessary to fully understand the long-term effects and optimize the cost-effectiveness of these therapies [63, 67].

Lovo-cel offers promising outcomes for SCD patients, with substantial improvements in clinical and quality-of-life measures. However, its high cost and access challenges highlight the need for continued research and policy efforts to make these therapies more accessible globally.

2.6.4 EDIT-301

Recent developments in the clinical trials of EDIT-301 for treating SCD have shown promising results. EDIT-301 is an investigational gene-edited autologous hematopoietic stem cell therapy that targets the γ-globin gene HBG1/HBG2 promoters to reactivate HbF production, thereby reducing sickling of red blood cells [68]. The RUBY trial, a Phase I/II study, evaluates the safety, tolerability, and efficacy of EDIT-301 in patients with severe SCD. Preliminary results indicate successful engraftment and a rapid, sustained increase in total hemoglobin and HbF levels, with significant improvements in hemolysis markers and no reported VOEs in treated subjects [68]. The trial involves collecting autologous CD34+ hematopoietic stem cells, editing them using the AsCas12a enzyme, and reinfusing them into patients after myeloablative conditioning with busulfan. The safety profile of EDIT-301 is consistent with the conditioning regimen, with no serious adverse events related to the gene therapy itself [68]. These findings support further investigation of EDIT-301 as a potential curative treatment for SCD, offering an alternative to the currently limited curative option of allogeneic hematopoietic stem cell transplantation [20]. EDIT-301's use of AsCas12a represents a novel approach with potentially fewer off-target effects [63]. Despite these advancements, challenges remain, including the high cost of gene therapies and the need for long-term studies to assess their durability and safety [20, 63]. The ongoing RUBY trial and similar studies are critical for validating the clinical efficacy and safety of EDIT-301, potentially transforming the treatment paradigm for SCD patients [20, 68].

2.6.5 BEAM-101

BEAM-101, a therapy developed by Beam Therapeutics, is a notable example of these advancements. BEAM-101 employs base editing to introduce single-point mutations in the promoter regions of the γ1 and γ2 genes, which encode subunits of HbF.

This approach aims to reactivate HbF production, which can outcompete HbS and restore normal hemoglobin function, thereby alleviating SCD symptoms [69].

The BEAM-101 therapy is part of a broader trend in SCD treatment that includes innovative gene editing strategies. These strategies focus on either correcting the genetic mutation responsible for SCD or modulating the expression of genes that can mitigate the disease's effects. For instance, other therapies in development, such as those by CRISPR Therapeutics and Vertex, also aim to upregulate HbF levels through different genetic modifications [20, 69]. Despite the promise of these therapies, challenges remain. The high cost and complexity of gene therapies pose significant barriers to widespread adoption, particularly in resource-limited settings [69]. Additionally, while BEAM-101 and similar therapies show potential in preclinical models, their long-term efficacy and safety in humans are still under investigation [69]. While BEAM-101 and similar gene editing therapies hold significant promise, they are still in the clinical trial phase and face challenges related to delivery, cost, and accessibility, particularly in resource-limited settings [70].

BEAM-101 represents a promising development in the treatment of SCD, leveraging advanced gene editing techniques to potentially offer a curative approach. However, the success of such therapies will depend on overcoming logistical and financial challenges, as well as ensuring patient-centered trial designs to enhance participation and efficacy [69, 70].

2.7 Other novel therapeutics to treat SCD complications

2.7.1 L-glutamine [Endari]

Glutamine, a conditionally essential amino acid, plays a crucial role in nitrogen transport and serves as a precursor for the synthesis of vital biological molecules, including glutathione, nicotinamide adenine dinucleotide (NAD), and arginine. In SCD, elevated reactive oxygen species (ROS) levels lead to red blood cell membrane damage, and therapeutic strategies that enhance HbF production or augment substrates for antioxidant pathways may mitigate ROS effects, though the precise biochemical role of glutamine in this context remains inadequately elucidated [71].

Recent developments in the use of L-glutamine [Endari] for treating SCD have shown promising results in reducing acute complications, particularly VOCs. A randomized controlled trial demonstrated that L-glutamine significantly decreased the number and severity of VOCs and hospitalizations in children with SCD over a 24-week period, compared to standard care. Additionally, it improved cerebral arterial blood flow, suggesting potential benefits beyond VOC reduction [72]. Pharmacokinetic and pharmacodynamic analyses have provided insights into the mechanisms of L-glutamine. Although the exact mechanisms remain unclear, studies have shown that higher exposure to L-glutamine is associated with increased hemoglobin concentration, improved RBC deformability, and decreased reactive oxygen species in reticulocytes. These effects suggest that L-glutamine may enhance RBC function and reduce oxidative stress, which are critical in managing SCD complications [73]. Furthermore, a population pharmacokinetic study indicated that L-glutamine has rapid absorption and elimination, with no significant drug accumulation, allowing for flexible dosing regimens. The study also found that food intake does not significantly affect L-glutamine clearance, making it convenient for patients [74]. Additionally, while systematic reviews are underway to evaluate the broader effects of amino acids like L-glutamine on SCD pain management, more randomized clinical trials are needed to confirm these benefits and optimize dosing strategies [75]. In summary, L-glutamine shows potential as a therapeutic option for reducing VOCs and improving RBC function in SCD patients. However, further research is necessary to fully understand its mechanisms and optimize its clinical use [72–74].

2.7.2 Defibrotide

Defibrotide is a polydisperse oligonucleotide authorized for hepatic vaso-occlusive disease post-HSCT [76]. Recent developments in the use of defibrotide for treating patients with SCD, particularly those experiencing Acute Chest Syndrome (ACS), have shown promising results. A Phase II investigation assessed the safety and efficacy of defibrotide in pediatric and adolescent patients [aged 2–40 years] with SCD-related ACS, revealing its well-tolerated nature and a significant reduction in inflammatory biomarkers, indicating potential therapeutic advantages in addressing endothelial dysfunction associated with ACS [77].

While defibrotide demonstrates promise, the evolving landscape of SCD treatment is characterized by the emergence of innovative therapies, including gene therapies that may provide curative options [20]. However, the high costs and uncertain long-term effects of these treatments necessitate extensive research, particularly to assess the efficacy of defibrotide in addressing endothelial dysfunction within the broader therapeutic framework for SCD, which requires validation through large-scale, randomized clinical trials [77]. This ongoing research is crucial for developing comprehensive treatment strategies that improve patient outcomes and quality of life for those suffering from SCD.

2.7.3 ALXN1820

The complement system, an integral part of the immune response, triggers inflammatory reactions to combat infections, yet recent research indicates that heightened activation through the alternate pathway correlates with complications in SCD, such as VOCs, hemolysis, inflammation, organ damage, and delayed hemolytic transfusion reactions [78].

In particular, aberrant regulation of the C5b-9 membrane attack complex is associated with a substantial increase in sickle cell lysis [79]. This positions the complement system as a plausible therapeutic target for SCD. ALXN1820 is a humanized, bispecific variable heavy domain antibody that concurrently binds to human albumin and properdin [80]. This antibody specifically inhibits the activation of the complement alternate pathway and possesses an extended circulatory half-life attributed to its interaction with albumin. Studies utilizing murine models have indicated that the inhibition of properdin leads to a significant reduction in VOCs and hemolysis, rendering ALXN1820 a promising novel therapeutic option [80]. The PHOENIX trial (NCT05565092) is a current phase 2a investigation assessing the safety and efficacy of ALXN1820 in adult populations affected by SCD. The primary endpoint of this study is the incidence of adverse treatment effects and serious adverse events; however, pharmacokinetics, alterations in baseline complement activation, hemoglobin levels, and hemolysis will also be evaluated.

2.7.4 Crovalimab

Crovalimab is a novel anti-complement C5 monoclonal antibody designed for subcutaneous administration, which targets complement dysregulation implicated in the pathophysiology of SCD, including vaso-occlusion, hemolysis, and inflammation [77].

The CROSSWALK-a trial, a Phase 1b investigation, assesses the safety profile of crovalimab in treating acute uncomplicated VOEs in patients aged 12–55 years with confirmed SCD [81]. Concurrently, the CROSSWALK-c trial, a Phase 2a study, evaluates the efficacy of crovalimab as an adjunct therapy for VOE prevention in patients experiencing multiple VOEs annually [82]. The ongoing research into crovalimab, with its promising safety and efficacy profile demonstrated in other complement-mediated disorders like paroxysmal nocturnal hemoglobinuria, suggests potential benefits for SCD patients [82]. However, the trials are still in progress, and their outcomes will be crucial in determining crovalimab's role in SCD management.

2.7.5 RNA aptamers

RNA aptamers are small, non-coding RNAs that can bind to specific targets with high affinity and specificity, similar to antibodies, and are identified through the SELEX process [83]. A notable advancement in the treatment of SCD is the discovery of RNA aptamers that effectively bind to sickle hemoglobin, thereby inhibiting its polymerization, which is pivotal in the disease's pathophysiology. The aptamers DE3A and OX3B demonstrate potential therapeutic value by prolonging polymerization delay and reducing HbS polymerization rates, with ongoing clinical trials assessing the broader application of aptamers in various hematologic disorders [84].

The efficacy of aptamers as therapeutic agents lies in their capacity to inhibit and modulate target proteins, positioning them as viable options for targeted drug delivery in diverse diseases. While RNA aptamers show promise, alternative strategies, including the induction of HbF via genetic and pharmacological methods, are also under investigation. These approaches target the amelioration of SCD symptoms by reactivating HBG gene expression, though efficacy and specificity challenges persist. In summary, RNA aptamers provide a novel avenue for SCD treatment, particularly by inhibiting HbS polymerization [84, 85]. Continued research and clinical evaluations are essential to assess their effectiveness and potential incorporation into standard SCD treatment protocols.

2.7.6 Nitric oxide modulation

Recent developments in nitric oxide (NO) therapies for treating SCD have focused on addressing the reduced bioavailability of NO, which is implicated in the pathogenesis of SCD-related complications such as VOCs and priapism. NO is a critical vasodilator that helps prevent the adhesion of sickled red blood cells to the endothelium and controls platelet aggregation, thereby reducing the risk of thrombus formation and associated complications like stroke and pulmonary embolism [86]. Innovative approaches include the synthesis of NO-releasing compounds, such as the aromatic aldehyde derivatives TD7-NO and VZHE039-NO. These compounds have shown promise in preclinical studies by releasing NO in vitro and in vivo, with VZHE039-NO demonstrating significant anti-adhesion properties relevant to VOEs [87]. This suggests potential for these compounds to mitigate some of the vascular complications of SCD. In the context of SCD-associated priapism, research has highlighted the dysfunction of the NO-cGMP-PDE5 pathway as a key mechanism. Therapeutic strategies targeting this pathway, including PDE5 inhibitors and NO donors, have shown promise in preclinical models. However, despite these advances, large clinical trials aimed at increasing NO bioavailability have not consistently demonstrated significant improvements in the frequency or duration of acute pain crises in SCD patients [87].

This suggests that while NO plays a role in SCD pathophysiology, its therapeutic potential may be limited by complex interactions in pain signaling pathways. Overall, while NO-based therapies offer potential benefits in managing SCD complications, further research is needed to fully understand the mechanisms of NO depletion and its role in SCD. This will aid in developing more effective treatment strategies that can be integrated with existing and emerging therapies, such as gene therapies, to improve patient outcomes [20].

2.7.7 Prasugrel

Prasugrel, an oral thienopyridine, irreversibly inhibits P2Y12 receptors, thus diminishing ADP-dependent platelet activation, which is pivotal in the pathophysiology of SCD related to platelet activation and vaso-occlusion [88]. Despite its well-tolerated profile and some attenuation of platelet activation, clinical trials including the DOVE trial have not substantiated its efficacy in significantly reducing VOCs or related events in pediatric SCD populations [89]. Nevertheless, findings from a multicenter multinational phase 3 clinical trial with 341 pediatric SCD patients indicated no marked reduction in vaso-occlusive pain events [90]. These inconclusive results underscore the intricate nature of SCD and indicate that further investigation is warranted to elucidate prasugrel's therapeutic potential and efficacy across diverse patient demographics.

3. Conclusion

In conclusion, various novel treatments for SCD have recently emerged. Hydroxyurea, a long-standing conventional treatment, effectively alleviates SCD-related pain but is associated with side effects and unclear mechanisms of action. Recently FDA-approved treatments, including voxelotor, crizanlizumab, and L-glutamine, effectively reduce vaso-occlusive crises and enhance SCD patients' quality of life, expanding therapeutic options. Stem cell transplantation is currently the sole curative option for SCD, though its application is constrained by associated risks and developmental challenges. Gene therapy has exhibited promising outcomes, warranting further studies and clinical trials to assess its efficacy and safety, thus offering hope for future curative interventions.

Author details

Mohammed Abdulwahid Almorish[1]* and Ali A. Alyahawi[2]

1 Laboratory Hematology and Immunohematology, Department of Hematology, Faculty of Medicine and Health Sciences, Sana'a University, Sana'a, Yemen

2 Faculty of Medical Sciences, Saba University, Sana'a, Yemen

*Address all correspondence to: m.almorish@su.edu.ye and almorish70@gmail.com

References

[1] Higgs DR, Wood WG. Genetic complexity in sickle cell disease. Proceedings of the National Academy of Sciences of the United States of America. 2008;**105**(33):11595-11596

[2] Brugnara C. Sickle cell dehydration: Pathophysiology and therapeutic applications. Clinical Hemorheology and Microcirculation. 2018;**68**(2-3):187-204

[3] Conran N, Franco-Penteado CF, Costa FF. Newer aspects of the pathophysiology of sickle cell disease vaso-occlusion. Hemoglobin. 2009;**33**(1):1-16

[4] Chakravorty S, Williams TN. Sickle cell disease: A neglected chronic disease of increasing global health importance. Archives of Disease in Childhood. 2015;**100**(1):48-53

[5] Lubeck D, Agodoa I, Bhakta N, Danese M, Pappu K, Howard R, et al. Estimated life expectancy and income of patients with sickle cell disease compared with those without sickle cell disease. JAMA Network Open. 2019;**2**(11):e1915374

[6] Schnog JB, Duits AJ, Muskiet FA, ten Cate H, Rojer RA, Brandjes DP. Sickle cell disease; a general overview. The Netherlands Journal of Medicine. 2004;**62**(10):364-374

[7] Tanhehco YC, Nathu G, Vasovic LV. Development of curative therapies for sickle cell disease. Frontiers in Medicine. 2022;**9**:1055540

[8] Lewis J, Guilcher GMT, Greenway SC. Reviewing the impact of hydroxyurea on DNA methylation and its potential clinical implications in sickle cell disease. European Journal of Haematology. 2024;**113**(3):264-272

[9] Casella JF, Furstenau DK, Adams RJ, Brambilla DJ, Lebensburger JD, Fehr JJ, et al. Hydroxyurea to prevent brain injury in children with sickle cell disease (HU Prevent)—A randomized, placebo-controlled phase II feasibility/pilot study. American Journal of Hematology. 2024;**99**(10):1906-1916. DOI: 10.1002/ajh.27423

[10] Nkya S, Nzunda C, Saukiwa E, Kaywanga F, Buchard E, Solometal D. Exploring pharmacogenetic factors influencing hydroxyurea response in tanzanian sickle cell disease patients: A genomic medicine approach. bioRxiv. 2024. DOI: 10.1101/2024.05.23.595488

[11] Diesch-Furlanetto T, Sanchez C, Atkinson A, Pondarré C, Dhedin N, Neven B, et al. Impact of hydroxyurea on follicle density in patients with sickle cell disease. Blood Advances. 2024;**8**(19):5227-5235. DOI: 10.1182/bloodadvances.2023011536

[12] Roessner C, Sale T, Uminski K, Goodyear D, Rydz N. A pharmacist-managed hydroxyurea prescribing protocol improves uptake and optimization among patients with sickle cell disease. Advances in Hematology. 2024;**2024**:4753349

[13] Saunthararajah Y, Woost PG, Friedrich U, Clausen WHO, Jacobberger JW, Lau H. 5613127 pharmacokinetics and pharmacodynamics of an innovative oral formulation of decitabine and tetrahydrouridine in healthy people. Hemasphere. 2023;7(Suppl.):16

[14] Molokie R, Lavelle D, Gowhari M, Pacini M, Krauz L, Hassan J, et al. Oral

tetrahydrouridine and decitabine for non-cytotoxic epigenetic gene regulation in sickle cell disease: A randomized phase 1 study. PLoS Medicine. 2017;**14**(9):e1002382

[15] Shearstone JR, Golonzhka O, Chonkar A, Tamang D, van Duzer JH, Jones SS, et al. Chemical inhibition of histone deacetylases 1 and 2 induces fetal hemoglobin through activation of GATA2. PLoS ONE. 2016;**11**(4):e0153767

[16] Esrick EB, McConkey M, Lin K, Frisbee A, Ebert BL. Inactivation of HDAC1 or HDAC2 induces gamma globin expression without altering cell cycle or proliferation. American Journal of Hematology. 2015;**90**(7):624-628

[17] Bradner JE, Mak R, Tanguturi SK, Mazitschek R, Haggarty SJ, Ross K, et al. Chemical genetic strategy identifies histone deacetylase 1 (HDAC1) and HDAC2 as therapeutic targets in sickle cell disease. Proceedings of the National Academy of Sciences of the United States of America. 2010;**107**(28):12617-12622

[18] Santos MEHP, Olops L, Vendrame F, Tavares AHJ, Leonardo DP, de Azevedo PC, et al. Benserazide as a potential novel fetal hemoglobin inducer: An observational study in non-carriers of hemoglobin disorders. Blood Cells, Molecules & Diseases. 2021;**87**:102511

[19] Pace BS, Perrine S, Li B, Makala L, Xu H, Takezaki M, et al. Benserazide racemate and enantiomers induce fetal globin gene expression in vivo: Studies to guide clinical development for beta thalassemia and sickle cell disease. Blood Cells, Molecules & Diseases. 2021;**89**:102561

[20] Barak M, Hu C, Matthews A, Fortenberry YM. Current and future therapeutics for treating patients with sickle cell disease. Cells. 2024;**13**(10):848

[21] Shah N, Andemariam B, Billett HH, Ershler WB, Bergmann S, Sakhalkar VS, et al. Voxelotor for sickle cell disease: Initial report from the real-world PROSPECT study. Journal of Sickle Cell Disease. 2024;**1**(Supplement. 1):yoae002.001

[22] Chaturvedi P, Shah SR. Assessing the clinical outcomes of voxelotor treatment in patients with sickle cell disease. International Journal of Applied Sciences and Biotechnology. 2024;**12**(1):46-53

[23] Brown C, Davis M, Achebe MO, Hassab H, Al-Kindi S, Telfer P, et al. Over 4 years of safety and efficacy with voxelotor in patients with sickle cell disease. Journal of Sickle Cell Disease. 2024;**1**(1):yoae002.008. DOI: 10.1093/jscdis/yoae002.008

[24] Muneeb Ansari X, Zhang IR, Farooqui M. Incidence of thromboembolic events in patients with sickle cell disease taking voxelotor. Journal of Sickle Cell Disease. 2024;**1**(Supplement. 1):yoae002.0152024

[25] Brothers RO, Turrentine KB, Akbar M, Triplett S, Zhao H, Urner TM, et al. The influence of voxelotor on cerebral blood flow and oxygen extraction in pediatric sickle cell disease. Blood. 2024;**143**(21):2145-2151

[26] Saraf SL, Abdullahi SU, Akinsete AM, Fasola FA, Idowu M, Pennington S, et al. Preliminary results from a multicenter phase 2/3 study of next-generation HbS polymerization inhibitor GBT021601 for the treatment of patients with sickle cell disease. Blood. 2023;**142**(Supplement. 1):274

[27] Pochron MP, Akinsete AM, Abdullahi SU, Fasola FA, Idowu M, Pennington S, et al. Preliminary pharmacodynamic results from a multicenter phase 2/3 study of next-generation HbS polymerization inhibitor GBT021601 for the treatment of patients with sickle cell disease. Blood. 2023;**142**(Supplement. 1):1155

[28] Pochron MP, Sun J, Potdar AA, Alt C, DeGuzman F, Connor MW, et al. Predictive biomarker analysis from the GBT021601 survival study in Townes sickle mice. Blood. 2023;**142**(Supplement. 1):14

[29] Dufu K, Alt C, Strutt S, Partridge J, Tang T, Siu V, et al. GBT021601 improves red blood cell health and the pathophysiology of sickle cell disease in a murine model. British Journal of Haematology. 2023;**202**(1):173-183

[30] van Dijk MJ, Ruiter TJJ, van der Veen S, Rab MAE, van Oirschot BA, Bos J, et al. Metabolic blood profile and response to treatment with the pyruvate kinase activator mitapivat in patients with sickle cell disease. HemaSphere. 2024;**8**(6):e109

[31] D'Alessandro A, Le K, Lundt M, Li Q, Dunkelberger EB, Cellmer T, et al. Functional and multi-omics signatures of mitapivat efficacy upon activation of pyruvate kinase in red blood cells from patients with sickle cell disease. Haematologica. 2024;**109**(8):2639-2652

[32] Conrey A, Frey I, Asomaning N, Charles RP, et al. Long-term safety and efficacy of mitapivat, an oral pyruvate kinase activator, in adults with sickle cell disease: Extension of a phase 1 dose escalation study. Blood. 2023;**142**(1):273. DOI: 10.1182/blood-2023-180165

[33] Jonassaint CR, Eppinger BA, Friend D, Green GL, Robinson M, Woolford T, et al. A patient-centric approach to sickle cell disease clinical trials: Integrating patient perspectives in the RISE UP phase 2/3 trial of mitapivat for informed protocol design and associated patient community benefit. Blood. 2023;**142**(Supplement. 1):2376

[34] Saraf SL, Hagar R, Idowu M, Osunkwo I, Cruz K, Kuypers FA, et al. Multicenter, phase 1 study of etavopivat (FT-4202) treatment for up to 12 weeks in patients with sickle cell disease. Blood Advances. 2024;**8**(16):4459-4475. DOI: 10.1182/bloodadvances.2023012467

[35] Telen M, Brown R, Hagar R, Idowu M, Osunkwo I, Kalfa T, et al. O-03: Etavopivat treatment for up to 12 weeks in patients with sickle cell disease is well tolerated and improves red blood cell health. Hema. 2022;**6**(Suppl.):02-03

[36] Colombatti R, Kanter J, Wu E, Clay LJ, Campbell A. Pb2524: Trial in progress: The hibiscus-kids study, a single-arm, open-label, phase 1/2 study to evaluate the pharmacokinetics and safety of etavopivat in pediatric patients with sickle cell disease. HemaSphere. 2023;**7**(S3):e544958a

[37] Schroeder P, Fulzele K, Forsyth S, Ribadeneira MD, Guichard S, Wilker E, et al. Etavopivat, a pyruvate kinase activator in red blood cells, for the treatment of sickle cell disease. The Journal of Pharmacology and Experimental Therapeutics. 2022;**380**(3):210-219

[38] Saraf S, Brown RC, Hagar RW, Idowu M, Osunkwo I, Kalfa TA, et al. P1495: Etavopivat treatment for up to 12 weeks in patients with sickle cell disease is well tolerated and improves red blood cell health. HemaSphere. 2022;**6**:1377-1378

[39] Poppenborg F, Röth A, Yamamoto R, Reinhardt HC, Alashkar F.

Crizanlizumab in adult patients with sickle cell disease: A retrospective German analysis. Frontiers in Hematology. 2024;**3**:1374181

[40] Abboud MR, Cançado RD, De Montalembert M, Smith WR, Rimawi H, Voskaridou E, et al. Efficacy, safety, and biomarker analysis of 5 mg and 7.5 mg doses of crizanlizumab in patients with sickle cell disease: Primary analyses from the phase III STAND study. Blood. 2023;**142**(Supplement. 1):272

[41] Kanter J, Brown RC, Norris C, Nair SM, Kutlar A, Manwani D, et al. Pharmacokinetics, pharmacodynamics, safety, and efficacy of crizanlizumab in patients with sickle cell disease. Blood Advances. 2023;**7**(6):943-952

[42] Chan KH, Buddharaju R, Idowu M. Real-world experience of patients with sickle cell disease treated with crizanlizumab. Journal of Investigative Medicine: The Official Publication of the American Federation for Clinical Research. 2024;**72**(2):242-247

[43] Abdulgayoom M, Afana MS, Alshurafa A, Yassin MA. Potential efficacy of crizanlizumab in treating priapism in sickle cell disease: A case report. Clinical Case Reports. 2024;**12**(5):e8585

[44] Mattè A, Federti E, Recchiuti A, Hamza M, Ferri G, Riccardi V, et al. Epeleuton, a novel synthetic ω-3 fatty acid, reduces hypoxia/reperfusion stress in a mouse model of sickle cell disease. Haematologica. 2024;**109**(6):1918-1932

[45] Andemariam B, Sheehan VA, Hamza M, Kelly K, Climax J. A phase 2, open-label study to assess the pharmacokinetics, pharmacodynamics and safety of orally administered epeleuton in patients with sickle cell disease. Blood. 2023;**142**(Supplement. 1):1159

[46] Hamza M, Downes B, Federici C, Braxton S, Sertel S, Combs G, et al. P1439: Epeleuton, a novel synthetic ω-3 fatty acid, reduces endothelial adhesion of red blood cells from sickle cell disease patients under physiological flow conditions. HemaSphere. 2023;**7**(S3):e599606f

[47] Allali S, Marquant F, Rignault-Bricard R, Taylor M, Brice J, de Montalembert M, et al. Oral famotidine reduces the plasma level of soluble P-selectin in children with sickle cell disease. British Journal of Haematology. 2024;**204**(1):346-351

[48] Andemariam B, Inati A, Colombatti R, Minniti C, Brown C, Hottmann M, et al. 5572697 trials in progress: The thrive studies evaluating the efficacy, safety, and long-term treatment with inclacumab, a p-selectin inhibitor, in patients with sickle cell disease. HemaSphere. 2023;**7**(S1):23-24

[49] Andemariam B, Inati A, Colombatti R, Minniti C, Brown C, Hottmann M, et al. P1486: Trials in progress: The thrive studies evaluating the efficacy, safety, and long-term treatment with inclacumab, a p-selectin inhibitor, in patients with sickle cell disease. HemaSphere. 2022;**6**:1368-1369

[50] Tarasev M, Herppich A, Gao X. Hines, S107: p-selectin inhibitor inclacumab reduces cell adhesion in an in-vitro assays showing potential for prevention of vaso-occlusion events in sickle cell disease. HemaSphere. 2022;**6**:3-4

[51] Manwani D, Chen G, Carullo V, Serban S, Olowokure O, Jang J, et al. Single-dose intravenous gammaglobulin can stabilize neutrophil mac-1 activation

in sickle cell pain crisis. American Journal of Hematology. 2015;**90**:381-385

[52] Manwani D, Xu C, Lee SK, Amatuni G, Cohen HW, Carullo V, et al. Randomized phase 2 trial of intravenous gamma globulin (IVIG) for the treatment of acute vaso-occlusive crisis in patients with sickle cell disease: Lessons learned from the midpoint analysis. Complementary Therapies in Medicine. 2020;**52**:102481

[53] AbuSamra DB, Aleisa FA, Al-Amoodi AS, Ahmed HMJ, Chin CJ, Abuelela AF, et al. Not just a marker: CD34 on human hematopoietic stem/progenitor cells dominates vascular selectin binding along with CD44. Blood Advances. 2017;**1**:2799-2816

[54] Esrick EB, Lehmann LE, Biffi A, Achebe M, Brendel C, Ciuculescu MF, et al. Post-transcriptional genetic silencing of BCL11A to treat sickle cell disease. The New England Journal of Medicine. 2021;**384**:205-215

[55] Salinas Cisneros G, Thein SL. Recent advances in the treatment of sickle cell disease. Frontiers in Physiology. 2020;**11**:435

[56] Brendel C, Negre O, Rothe M, Guda S, Parsons G, Harris C, et al. Preclinical evaluation of a novel lentiviral vector driving lineage-specific BCL11A knockdown for sickle cell gene therapy. Molecular Therapy - Methods & Clinical Development. 2020;**17**:589-600

[57] Zarghamian P, Klermund J, Cathomen T. Clinical genome editing to treat sickle cell disease—A brief update. Frontiers in Medicine. 2023;**9**:1065377

[58] Frangoul H, Locatelli F, Sharma A, Bhatia M, Mapara M, Molinari L, et al. Exagamglogene autotemcel for severe sickle cell disease. The New England Journal of Medicine. 2024;**390**(18):1649-1662

[59] Frangoul H, Locatelli F, Sharma A, Bhatia M, Mapara MY, Molinari L, et al. Elimination of vaso-occlusive crises after exagamglogene autotemcel in patients with severe sickle cell disease. Transplantation and Cellular Therapy. 2024;**30**(2):S234-S235

[60] Singh A, Irfan H, Fatima E, Nazir Z, Verma A, Akilimali A. Revolutionary breakthrough: FDA approves CASGEVY, the first CRISPR/Cas9 gene therapy for sickle cell disease. Annals of Medicine and Surgery. 2024;**86**(8):4555-4559

[61] Mohammadian Gol T, Zahedipour F, Trosien P, Ureña-Bailén G, Kim M, Antony JS, et al. Gene therapy in pediatrics—Clinical studies and approved drugs (as of 2023). Life Sciences. 2024;**348**:122685

[62] Adashi EY, Gruppuso PA, Cohen IG. CRISPR therapy of sickle cell disease: The dawning of the gene editing era. The American Journal of Medicine. 2024;**137**(5):390-392

[63] Leonard A, Tisdale JF. A new frontier: FDA approvals for gene therapy in sickle cell disease. Molecular Therapy: The Journal of the American Society of Gene Therapy. 2024;**32**(2):264-267

[64] Ashinze P. Revolutionizing sickle cell disease treatment: Unveiling CRISPR and lentiviral therapies—Navigating complexities in access, equity, and global health dynamics. Plasmatology. 2024;**18**. DOI: 10.1177/26348535241254682

[65] Kanter J, Thompson AA, Kwiatkowski JL, Parikh SH, Mapara M, Rifkin-Zenenberg S, et al. Efficacy, safety, and health-related quality of life (HRQOL) in patients with SCD who have received lovotibeglogene

autotemcel (Lovo-cel) gene therapy: Up to 60 months of follow-up. Blood. 2023;**142**(Supplement 1):1051. DOI: 10.1182/blood-2023-174229

[66] Herring WL, Gallagher ME, Shah N, Morse KC, Mladsi D, Dong OM, et al. Cost-effectiveness of lovotibeglogene autotemcel (Lovo-Cel) gene therapy for patients with sickle cell disease and recurrent vaso-occlusive events in the United States. PharmacoEconomics. 2024;**42**(6):693-714

[67] Nikitin D, Beaudoin FL, Thokala P, McKenna A, Nhan E, Rind DM, et al. Gene therapies for sickle cell disease: Effectiveness and value. Journal of Managed Care & Specialty Pharmacy. 2023;**29**(11):1253-1259

[68] Hanna R, Frangoul H, Mckinney C, Pineiro L, Mapara M, Chang KH, et al. S264: Edit-301 shows promising preliminary safety and efficacy results in the phase i/ii clinical trial (ruby) of patients with severe sickle cell disease using highly specific and efficient ascas12a enzyme. HemaSphere. 2023;**7**(Suppl.):e05170e0

[69] Sarkar AA. The current state of sickle cell disease treatments. GEN Biotechnology. 2022;**1**(6):565-571

[70] Liang H, Yang G, Yang Z, Luo Z. Innovation method to deliver gene editor ABE to treat sickle cell disease by nanotechnology combined with DNA origami. Academic Journal of Medicine & Health Sciences. 2024;**5**(6):45-54

[71] Sadaf A, Quinn CT. L-glutamine for sickle cell disease: Knight or pawn? Experimental Biology and Medicine. 2020;**245**:146-154

[72] Ebeid FSE, Aly NH, Shaheen NM, Abdellatif SMA, Okba AAM, Gad NA, et al. Safety and efficacy of L-glutamine in reducing the frequency of acute complications among patients with sickle cell disease: A randomized controlled study. Annals of Hematology. 2024;**103**:3493-3506. DOI: 10.1007/s00277-024-05877-8

[73] Sadaf A, Dong M, Pfeiffer A, Korpik J, Kalfa TA, Latham T, et al. A pharmacokinetic-pharmacodynamic analysis of l-glutamine for the treatment of sickle cell disease: Implications for understanding the mechanism of action and evaluating response to therapy. British Journal of Haematology. 2024;**205**(3):1147-1158. DOI: 10.1111/bjh.19632

[74] Sadaf A, Dong M, Pfeiffer A, Latham T, Kalfa T, Vinks AA, et al. A population pharmacokinetic analysis of L-glutamine exposure in patients with sickle cell disease: Evaluation of dose and food effects. Clinical Pharmacokinetics. 2024;**63**(3):357-365

[75] Sadaf A, Dong M, Korpik J, Pfeiffer A, Kalfa TA, Latham TS, et al. Effects of L-glutamine on biomarkers of response in sickle cell disease: A pharmacokinetics-pharmacodynamics analysis. Blood. 2023;**142**(Supplement. 1):1145

[76] Baker DE, Demaris K. Defibrotide. Hospital Pharmacy. 2016;**51**:847-854

[77] Schaefer E, Kanarfogel T, Hochberg JC, Thatcher E, Klejmont L, Chu Y, et al. A phase II study to evaluate the safety and efficacy of defibrotide in sickle cell disease-related acute chest syndrome (IND 127812). Blood. 2022;**140**(Supplement. 1):2532-2534

[78] Varelas C, Tampaki A, Sakellari I, Anagnostopoulos A, Gavriilaki E, Vlachaki E. Complement in sickle cell disease: Are we ready for prime

time? Journal of Blood Medicine. 2021;**12**:177-187

[79] Tampaki A, Gavriilaki E, Varelas C, Anagnostopoulos A, Vlachaki E. Complement in sickle cell disease and targeted therapy: I know one thing, that I know nothing. Blood Reviews. 2021;**48**:100805

[80] Dai Y, Hill K, Harris D, Shen T, Yuan C-X, Gasteyger C. A phase 2a, randomized, open-label study to evaluate multiple dosing regimens of subcutaneous ALXN1820 in adult patients with sickle cell disease. Blood. 2022;**140**:8298-8299

[81] Bartolucci P, Ataga KI, Callaghan M, De Franceschi L, Minniti C, Alexandrou A, et al. 5610823 trial in progress: The randomized, double-blind, placebo-controlled phase 1b crosswalk-a trial evaluating the safety of crovalimab for the management of acute uncomplicated vaso-occlusive episodes (VOES) in patients (PTS) with sickle cell disease (SCD). HemaSphere. 2023;**7**(Suppl.):22

[82] Callaghan M, Ataga K, De Franceschi L, Minniti C, Balachandran N, Imbs D, et al. P120: The trail in progress: The randomized, double-blind, placebo-controlled phase 2A crosswalk-C trial evaluating crovalimab as adjunct treatment in the prevention of vaso-occlusive episodes in patients with sickle cell disease (SCD). HemaSphere. 2022;**6**(Suppl.):27-28

[83] Li Y, Wu H, Niu Y, Hu Y, Li Q, Cao C, et al. Development of RNA aptamer-based therapeutic agents. Current Medicinal Chemistry. 2013;**20**(29):3655-3663

[84] Purvis SH, Keefer JR, Fortenberry YM, Barron-Casella EA, Casella JF. Identification of aptamers that bind to sickle hemoglobin and inhibit its polymerization. Nucleic Acid Therapeutics. 2017;**27**(6):354-364

[85] Starlard-Davenport A, Gu Q, Pace BS. Targeting genetic modifiers of HBG gene expression in sickle cell disease: The miRNA option. Molecular Diagnosis & Therapy. 2022;**26**(5):497-509

[86] Gupta P, Kumar R. Nitric oxide: A potential etiological agent for vaso-occlusive crises in sickle cell disease. Nitric Oxide: Biology and Chemistry. 2024;**144**:40-46

[87] Pereira DA, Calmasini FB, Costa FF, Burnett AL, Silva FH. Nitric oxide resistance in priapism associated with sickle cell disease: Mechanisms, therapeutic challenges, and future directions. The Journal of Pharmacology and Experimental Therapeutics. 2024;**390**(2):203-212

[88] Moser BA, LaBell ES, Chigutsa E, Jakubowski JA, Small DS. Population pharmacokinetic and exposure-response analyses of prasugrel in pediatric patients with sickle cell anemia. Clinical Pharmacokinetics. 2018;**57**(2):243-254

[89] Heeney MM, Hoppe CC, Rees DC. Prasugrel for sickle cell vaso-occlusive events. The New England Journal of Medicine. 2016;**375**(2):185-186

[90] Heeney MM, Hoppe CC, Abboud MR, Inusa B, Kanter J, Ogutu B, et al. A multinational trial of prasugrel for sickle cell vaso-occlusive events. The New England Journal of Medicine. 2016;**374**:625-635

Chapter 4

Perspective Chapter: Advances in Diagnosis of Beta Thalassemia Major

Zeynep Ece Demirbaş

Abstract

Beta Thalassemia Major is a severe inherited blood disorder caused by mutations in the HBB gene, resulting in reduced or absent production of beta-globin chains. This condition leads to chronic anemia, requiring regular blood transfusions and iron chelation therapy. The disorder is prevalent in regions such as the Mediterranean, Middle East, South Asia, and Southeast Asia. Advances in molecular diagnostics, including PCR and non-invasive prenatal testing, have significantly improved early detection and treatment outcomes. Screening and prevention programs in high-risk areas have reduced the number of affected births. The use of artificial intelligence in specific diagnostic areas, particularly in managing iron overload, is also being explored to enhance patient care. This chapter covers the genetic structure, clinical manifestations, diagnostic methods, and iron overload management in Beta Thalassemia Major.

Keywords: beta thalassemia major, hemoglobinopathies, molecular diagnostics, iron overload, artificial intelligence, prenatal screening, blood transfusion

1. Introduction

Beta Thalassemia Major (BTM) is an inherited blood disorder caused by mutations in the HBB gene, which leads to reduced or absent production of the beta-globin chains of hemoglobin. As a result, patients experience severe microcytic anemia, which requires lifelong medical management including blood transfusions and iron chelation therapy.

1.1 Prevalence

Beta Thalassemia is one of the most common monogenic disorders worldwide, with particularly high prevalence in regions known as the "thalassemia belt," which includes parts of the Mediterranean, Middle East, South Asia, and Southeast Asia. Globally, it is estimated that 1.5–5% of the population are carriers of beta thalassemia [1]. In Mediterranean countries like Italy and Greece, the carrier rate can reach up to 10%. In parts of the Indian subcontinent, particularly in India and Pakistan, the carrier rate is about 3–4%. Southeast Asia, including countries like Thailand and Malaysia, also has a significant carrier rate, estimated between 4 and 6% [2].

In Turkey, the national carrier rate is estimated to be around 4%, with some regions showing much higher frequencies due to historical genetic flow and population migrations [3]. Every year, approximately 60,000–100,000 children are born with severe forms of thalassemia, including BTM [1].

2. Genetic structure and pathophysiology

Beta Thalassemia Major results from mutations in the HBB gene, which encodes the beta-globin chain of hemoglobin. The normal adult hemoglobin (HbA) molecule consists of two alpha and two beta-globin chains [4]. In BTM, mutations lead to the reduction or absence of beta-globin chain production, which disrupts normal hemoglobin synthesis and causes ineffective erythropoiesis [5].

2.1 Genetic mutations in beta thalassemia

Beta thalassemia is primarily caused by over 200 different mutations in the HBB gene, ranging from point mutations to large deletions. These mutations are classified into two main types:

- β^0 *mutations:* These result in no production of beta-globin chains.
- β^+ *mutations:* These allow for reduced production of beta-globin chains.

Patients with BTM inherit two defective alleles (one from each parent), which can be either homozygous for β^0 or compound heterozygous for β^0/β^+ mutations [6].

2.2 Pathophysiology

The pathophysiology of BTM is characterized by:

- *Ineffective erythropoiesis:* The imbalance between alpha and beta chains leads to the formation of insoluble alpha-chain aggregates, which damage red blood cell (RBC) precursors in the bone marrow, resulting in premature destruction of these cells.
- *Hemolysis:* Red blood cells that escape the bone marrow enter circulation, but they are fragile and prone to destruction by the spleen, leading to hemolysis and worsening anemia.
- *Iron overload:* Due to frequent blood transfusions, patients develop secondary iron overload, particularly in organs such as the liver and heart. This can lead to complications like cardiomyopathy, liver cirrhosis, and endocrine dysfunction [7].

3. Traditional diagnostic methods

The diagnosis of BTM is typically confirmed through a combination of clinical presentation and hematological tests, with specific values that guide diagnosis [8].

- *Hemoglobin levels*: Patients with BTM usually exhibit severe microcytic anemia, with hemoglobin levels ranging between 3 and 4 g/dL.
- Hemoglobin Electrophoresis:
  - *HbA*: Reduced or absent in Beta Thalassemia Major, with HbA often below 5%.
  - *HbF*: Fetal hemoglobin (HbF) is elevated, constituting up to 95% of total hemoglobin.
  - *HbA2*: Typically absent in severe cases.
- *Mean corpuscular volume (MCV) and mean corpuscular hemoglobin (MCH)*: MCV is usually <70 fL, while MCH is often <27 pg.
- *Peripheral blood smear:* It commonly reveals target cells, microcytosis, hypochromia, and nucleated red blood cells.

4. Molecular diagnostic methods

Molecular diagnostics have revolutionized the detection and confirmation of BTM, allowing precise identification of genetic mutations in the HBB gene. The most widely used molecular method is Polymerase Chain Reaction (PCR), which amplifies specific DNA sequences to detect mutations responsible for beta thalassemia [9, 10]. There are several PCR-based techniques used for different diagnostic purposes:

4.1 Amplification refractory mutation system (ARMS-PCR)

ARMS-PCR is a highly specific PCR method designed to detect known point mutations in the HBB gene [11, 12]. This method is based on the selective amplification of mutant alleles, allowing for the differentiation between wild-type and mutated sequences. It is particularly useful for confirming specific known mutations in patients who are suspected carriers or affected by BTM.

Advantages: It is rapid, cost-effective, and suitable for screening populations with known mutation patterns.

4.2 Gap-PCR (deletion detection)

Gap-PCR is used for identifying deletions in the HBB gene region. Large deletions are a common cause of thalassemia syndromes, and Gap-PCR helps in detecting these deletions by amplifying across the breakpoints. It is commonly used in populations where large deletions are known to contribute to the disease [13, 14].

Advantages: This method is essential for detecting large structural variations that would be missed by other PCR techniques.

4.3 Real-time quantitative PCR (qPCR)

qPCR allows for the quantification of specific DNA sequences in real-time, making it useful for both diagnostic and research purposes. In the context of beta thalassemia, it is employed to quantify the relative expression of globin genes and assess gene copy numbers, which can provide insights into disease severity [15–17].

Advantages: High sensitivity, real-time data collection, and the ability to quantify gene expression or copy number changes.

4.4 Multiplex ligation-dependent probe amplification (MLPA)

MLPA is another PCR-based technique used to detect large deletions or duplications in the HBB gene and other genes involved in thalassemia. It can assess the copy number variations and is useful when combined with other PCR techniques for a comprehensive genetic diagnosis [18–22].

Advantages: Capable of detecting both small point mutations and larger structural changes.

4.5 Sanger sequencing (PCR-based)

Sanger sequencing is often used for direct mutation detection in the HBB gene. The PCR-amplified region of the gene is sequenced to detect any mutations or deletions. Sanger sequencing is highly accurate and is typically used when other methods fail to provide clear results, especially in identifying rare mutations [23].

Advantages: High accuracy and reliability in detecting both common and rare mutations.

4.6 Next-generation sequencing (NGS)

NGS is a more advanced molecular technique that allows for the parallel sequencing of multiple genes or regions of interest. In the context of beta thalassemia, NGS is increasingly being used for comprehensive mutation screening, including detecting rare mutations and compound heterozygosity. NGS can sequence the entire HBB gene and other associated genes simultaneously, providing a detailed genetic profile of the patient [24–26].

Advantages: High throughput, capable of identifying complex genetic variations, and provides detailed genetic information.

4.7 Non-invasive prenatal testing (NIPT) using PCR

NIPT for BTM involves analyzing fetal DNA present in maternal blood. PCR is used to amplify fetal DNA fragments to detect mutations in the HBB gene. This method is non-invasive and poses no risk to the fetus, making it an ideal option for prenatal diagnosis [27, 28].

Advantages: Safe, non-invasive, and provides early diagnostic results during pregnancy.

5. Iron overload in beta thalassemia major

Patients with BTM frequently undergo regular blood transfusions, which, while necessary to manage severe anemia, result in iron overload over time. Without adequate iron excretion, the body accumulates excess iron, leading to toxic deposits in various organs. This iron overload causes damage and dysfunction, particularly in the liver, heart, and endocrine glands.

5.1 Clinical manifestations of iron overload

Iron overload typically manifests in organs that store iron, leading to various clinical complications [1, 29, 30]:

- *Liver*: The liver is the primary site of iron storage, and iron overload here can cause hepatic fibrosis, cirrhosis, and even hepatocellular carcinoma if left untreated. Liver dysfunction often precedes more severe complications, making it critical to monitor iron levels in this organ.

- *Heart*: Iron deposition in the heart is one of the most serious complications of thalassemia. It can lead to cardiomyopathy, arrhythmias, and ultimately heart failure. Cardiac complications are the leading cause of death in patients with iron overload.

- *Endocrine glands*: Iron overload can damage various endocrine glands, leading to hypothyroidism, hypogonadism, diabetes mellitus, and growth failure. The pituitary, thyroid, pancreas, and gonads are commonly affected.

5.2 Organ involvement and screening protocols

To mitigate the effects of iron overload, regular screening and early detection are crucial. **Table 1** summarizes the key organs affected by iron overload, the complications associated with each, and the recommended screening frequency based on the severity of iron overload:

5.2.1 Liver involvement and screening

The liver is often the first organ to accumulate excess iron. Liver Iron Concentration (LIC) measured by MRI is the gold standard for detecting and quantifying hepatic iron overload [31–35]. Elevated LIC levels (greater than 7 mg Fe/g dry

Organ	Complications	Screening modality	Frequency
Liver	Hepatic fibrosis, cirrhosis, hepatocellular carcinoma	MRI (Liver Iron Concentration - LIC), Serum Ferritin	Every 6–12 months
Heart	Cardiomyopathy, arrhythmias, heart failure	MRI (Cardiac T2*), Echocardiogram	Annually (more frequently if LIC > 7 mg/g)
Endocrine Glands	Hypogonadism, hypothyroidism, diabetes mellitus	Serum hormone levels (TSH, LH, FSH, glucose)	Every 12 months (more frequent in severe cases)
Pancreas	Diabetes mellitus	Glucose tolerance test, HbA1c	Every 6–12 months
Spleen	Splenomegaly, hypersplenism	Ultrasound	Every 12 months (if spleen enlarged)
Bones	Osteoporosis, bone fractures	Bone density scan (DEXA), Vitamin D levels	Every 1–2 years

Table 1.
Organs affected by iron overload, complications associated with each and recommended screening frequnecy.

weight) indicate significant iron burden, increasing the risk of liver fibrosis and cirrhosis. Serum ferritin levels are also monitored as a marker of total body iron stores, but ferritin can be influenced by inflammation and infection [1, 36].

Recommended Screening: MRI to assess LIC every 6–12 months, and serum ferritin every 3–6 months in patients receiving regular transfusions [37–39].

5.2.2 Heart involvement and screening

Iron deposition in the heart can lead to serious complications, including cardiomyopathy and arrhythmias, which are the leading causes of mortality in BTM [40–42]. Cardiac T2 MRI* is a specialized imaging technique used to assess myocardial iron concentration. A T2 value less than 20 ms* suggests significant iron overload and the need for aggressive iron chelation therapy [1, 33, 43, 44].

Recommended Screening: Cardiac T2* MRI should be performed annually for early detection of myocardial iron overload, with more frequent monitoring in patients with LIC levels above 7 mg/g [45].

5.2.3 Endocrine complications and screening

Iron accumulation in endocrine organs can lead to a range of complications, including growth failure, delayed puberty, and hypothyroidism [46, 47]. Screening involves regular assessment of hormone levels:

- *Thyroid function:* Thyroid-stimulating hormone (TSH) and free T4 levels should be measured annually to detect hypothyroidism [1, 48].

- *Gonadal function:* In adolescents and adults, luteinizing hormone (LH) and follicle-stimulating hormone (FSH) levels are measured to assess for hypogonadism [49, 50].

- *Pancreatic function:* Glucose tolerance tests and HbA1c levels should be checked regularly to monitor for diabetes [51–53].

5.2.4 Bone health and screening

Patients with Beta Thalassemia Major are at increased risk for osteoporosis and fractures due to iron deposition in the bone marrow, along with vitamin D deficiency [54–57]. Dual-energy X-ray absorptiometry (DEXA) is used to assess bone density, and vitamin D levels are checked periodically.

Recommended Screening: DEXA scans every 1–2 years to monitor bone health, with more frequent scans if osteoporosis is diagnosed [1].

5.3 Management of iron overload

Managing iron overload involves the use of iron chelation therapy, with medications like Deferoxamine, Deferasirox, and Deferiprone used to promote iron excretion. The choice of chelator and the intensity of therapy depend on the severity of the iron burden, as determined by the screening protocols mentioned above. Chelation therapy aims to maintain LIC levels below 3 mg Fe/g dry weight and cardiac T2* above 20 ms to prevent complications [58, 59].

6. New diagnostic technologies

In recent years, advancements in diagnostic technologies have significantly improved the accuracy and speed of diagnosing BTM. These new methods offer more precise data, early detection, and non-invasive techniques, transforming how thalassemia is diagnosed and managed.

6.1 3 T magnetic resonance imaging (MRI)

MRI is a critical tool in assessing iron overload in patients with BTM, particularly in the liver and heart [33–35, 37, 60]. The 3 Tesla (3 T) MRI system has shown increased accuracy in quantifying iron deposition compared to earlier technologies. It is non-invasive and provides clear differentiation between organ tissues, making it ideal for monitoring iron accumulation and guiding chelation therapy [61–65].

LIC and cardiac iron concentration (T2)* are two key parameters measured via MRI to assess iron overload. Regular monitoring using 3 T MRI helps clinicians adjust treatment regimens accordingly.

6.2 Non-invasive prenatal diagnosis (NIPD)

Non-invasive prenatal testing (NIPT) is a breakthrough method for early detection of beta thalassemia during pregnancy [24, 66]. By analyzing *cell-free fetal DNA (cffDNA)* circulating in the maternal blood, NIPT allows for genetic screening without the risks associated with invasive procedures like amniocentesis or chorionic villus sampling (CVS) [67].

NIPT utilizes next-generation sequencing (NGS) or quantitative PCR to detect mutations in the HBB gene that cause beta thalassemia. The test can be conducted as early as the 7th to 9th week of pregnancy, offering an accurate and safe option for early prenatal diagnosis. Sensitivity and specificity rates for detecting common mutations have been reported to be over 99% in various studies [67].

While NIPT is highly effective for detecting common mutations in the HBB gene, rare or complex mutations may be missed, necessitating further testing and cost may remain a barrier particularly in low-resource settings [68].

Also, there can be challenges if the proportion of cffDNA is too low, particularly in early pregnancy or if gestational age is low [69].

6.3 Next-generation sequencing (NGS)

NGS has transformed genetic diagnostics by enabling the simultaneous sequencing of multiple regions of the genome, including the entire HBB gene [24, 70]. This method is particularly useful for identifying rare and complex mutations in beta thalassemia and provides a comprehensive genetic profile of the patient [71, 72].

NGS can also be applied in prenatal testing, providing a detailed view of potential mutations in both carriers and affected fetuses [70, 73].

6.4 Third-generation sequencing (TGS)

Third-generation sequencing (tgs) offers advantages over next-generation sequencing (NGS) in its ability to produce longer reads and more accurate haplotype phasing. This can be particularly beneficial in complex cases of thalassemia where copy number variations (CNVs) and rearrangements occur in genes like HBA and HBB. Including TGS as a tool for detecting rare mutations and structural variations would highlight the cutting-edge molecular approaches being adopted in thalassemia diagnosis.

TGS, especially with platforms like PacBio's SMRT and Oxford Nanopore Technologies (ONT), provides superior haplotype phasing, which allows for the detection of both common and rare mutations within the globin gene clusters. This level of precision is critical for genetic counseling and predicting disease severity in thalassemia patients [74–76].

6.5 Thermogravimetric analysis (TGA) and chemometrics for screening

This method provides a novel approach for diagnosing and classifying beta thalassemia by analyzing the thermal behavior of blood samples. It offers 100% accuracy in classification and is capable of distinguishing between different severities of thalassemia (e.g., TI-TD, TI-NTD, and TM-TD).

In TGA, a small sample of the patient's blood is gradually heated in a controlled environment. As the temperature increases, various components of the blood decompose at different rates, leading to changes in the sample's mass. These mass changes are recorded, and a thermogram (a plot of mass loss versus temperature) is generated. The patterns of thermal decomposition differ between normal, carrier, and affected individuals, allowing for clear distinction between these groups.

The analysis is typically supported by *chemometric methods*, which use statistical and computational techniques to interpret the complex data from TGA thermograms. The integration of TGA with chemometrics enhances the precision of the diagnosis, achieving a classification accuracy rate of nearly 100% in distinguishing between different thalassemia types and disease severities.

Advantages:

- *Non-invasive*: TGA only requires a small blood sample, which makes it less invasive compared to tissue biopsies or repeated genetic tests.

- *Rapid and accurate:* TGA, coupled with chemometrics, allows for rapid classification and diagnosis, reducing the need for more time-consuming molecular methods in some cases.

- *Cost-effective:* Since TGA relies on physical properties rather than expensive molecular diagnostics, it can potentially be a cost-effective option, particularly in regions with limited access to advanced genetic testing technologies.

The ability of TGA to accurately diagnose and classify beta thalassemia makes it a promising tool, especially in low-resource settings where conventional genetic testing may not be readily available. Its low-cost and non-invasive nature could enable more widespread screening and early diagnosis in high-prevalence regions like South Asia, the Mediterranean, and the Middle East [77, 78].

7. The role of artificial intelligence (AI) in diagnosis

Artificial intelligence (AI) has emerged as a valuable tool in the diagnosis, classification, and management of beta thalassemia major. AI algorithms, including machine learning (ML) models, have demonstrated the ability to accurately diagnose thalassemia and distinguish it from other forms of microcytic anemia, such as iron deficiency anemia (IDA), by analyzing large datasets and complex patterns within complete blood count (CBC) parameters.

7.1 AI in thalassemia diagnosis

AI systems are increasingly used to streamline the diagnostic process for thalassemia by automating the interpretation of laboratory data. These algorithms are designed to analyze hematological indices such as mean corpuscular volume (MCV), mean corpuscular hemoglobin (MCH), RBC distribution width (RDW), and hemoglobin electrophoresis results to differentiate between thalassemia and other causes of anemia [79].

Studies have demonstrated the use of several ML models, such as k-nearest neighbor (k-NN), Naïve Bayesian, and decision tree classifiers, to identify thalassemia carriers and patients with high accuracy. These models work by analyzing CBC data and other diagnostic parameters, achieving sensitivity and specificity values above 90% [79, 80].

Artificial Neural Networks (ANNs), which mimic the human brain's ability to process information, have shown even higher accuracy in diagnosing thalassemia. A study reported that ANNs achieved a sensitivity of 93.13% and specificity of 92.33% in discriminating between IDA and beta thalassemia [81–83].

7.2 AI for differentiation of thalassemia from other anemias

One of the key challenges in diagnosing thalassemia is distinguishing it from other forms of microcytic anemia, particularly IDA. AI models have been instrumental in addressing this diagnostic challenge:

AI models use hematological indices such as the Mentzer index, Green and King index, and others to differentiate between thalassemia and IDA [84, 85]. For instance, the Matos and Carvalho Index (MCI), which incorporates RBC count and MCHC values, was developed to improve differentiation, with a reported sensitivity of 99.3% [86].

Tools like ThalPred, developed using ML algorithms such as random forest and k-nearest neighbor, have made it easier for clinicians to diagnose thalassemia trait from IDA. These tools have achieved an accuracy of over 95% in clinical testing [87].

7.3 AI in iron overload management

Iron overload is a major complication in patients with transfusion-dependent thalassemia, and AI is being used to enhance the detection and management of iron deposition in critical organs such as the liver and heart.

AI algorithms have been integrated into MRI-based LIC assessments. A study developed a deep learning-based medical device to automate liver iron measurements using MRI. This model achieved sensitivity and specificity rates exceeding 90% in predicting LIC values [88].

AI systems also play a role in detecting iron overload in the heart using T2 MRI*. ML models analyze myocardial iron deposition and help clinicians make more accurate assessments of cardiac iron levels, reducing human error and improving treatment outcomes [89, 90].

7.4 AI in predicting thalassemia complications

AI has expanded beyond diagnosis to predict long-term complications in thalassemia patients, including organ damage from iron overload. By analyzing patient data over time, AI models can predict the likelihood of complications such as diabetes mellitus in thalassemia patients [91].

7.5 AI and decision support systems

AI-based clinical decision support systems (CDSS) are now being used to assist clinicians in making treatment decisions for thalassemia patients. These systems take into account a patient's genetic profile, transfusion history, and iron levels to recommend optimal treatment strategies, including iron chelation therapy. Such systems have been shown to reduce clinical decision errors and improve patient outcomes by providing data-driven recommendations [92–94].

The integration of AI into the diagnosis and management of BTM is revolutionizing the field by enhancing diagnostic accuracy, improving differentiation from other anemias, and aiding in the early detection of complications. As AI models become more sophisticated, their role in personalized medicine and real-time clinical decision-making will continue to grow, offering new opportunities for improving patient care.

8. Conclusions

BTM is a severe genetic disorder that imposes significant health challenges on affected individuals, particularly in regions with a high prevalence of hemoglobinopathies. Advances in both molecular diagnostic techniques, such as PCR and non-invasive prenatal testing, and imaging technologies like 3 Tesla MRI for iron overload monitoring, have greatly improved the management of the disease. Early detection through screening programs in high-risk populations has proven effective in reducing the incidence of BTM, offering hope for better patient outcomes and reduced healthcare burden.

Despite these advancements, the lifelong need for regular blood transfusions and the risk of iron overload remain critical concerns. The continuous development of chelation therapies and the integration of emerging technologies, such as AI, in both diagnostics and treatment monitoring hold promise for further enhancing patient care. Comprehensive, multidisciplinary approaches involving genetic counseling, preventive programs, and long-term management are essential in addressing the complexities of BTM. Continued research and collaboration at the global level will be key to improving the quality of life for patients with BTM.

Acknowledgements

The author would like to state that no external funding was received for this chapter. The work presented here was completed independently by the author, without additional contributions.

The author also acknowledges the use of ChatGPT 4.0 for language polishing of the manuscript.

Thanks

Thanks to my collogues for their valuable support. Their insights and expertise greatly enriched the development of this chapter.

Appendices and nomenclature

BTM	beta thalassemia major
HbA	adult hemoglobin (composed of two alpha and two beta chains)
HbF	fetal hemoglobin
HbA2	minor form of adult hemoglobin
PCR	polymerase chain reaction
LIC	liver iron concentration
HBB Gene	the gene responsible for encoding beta-globin chains
Alpha Chains	one of the two types of protein chains in normal hemoglobin
Beta Chains	the second type of protein chain in normal hemoglobin, deficient in beta thalassemia major

Author details

Zeynep Ece Demirbaş
Department of Internal Medicine, Dr. Siyami Ersek Thoracic and Cardiovascular Surgery Training and Research Hospital, Istanbul, Turkey

*Address all correspondence to: zeynepece@gmail.com

References

[1] Taher A, Musallam K, Cappellini MD. Guidelines for the Management of Non-transfusion-Dependent β-Thalassaemia. 3rd ed. Nicosia, Cyprus: Thalassaemia International Federation; 2023

[2] Bain A. Management of Transfusion Dependent Thalassaemia (TDT): A Short Guide. Thalass Int Fed Nicos Cyprus. 2022

[3] Canatan D, Kose MR, Ustundag M, Haznedaroglu D, Ozbas S. Hemoglobinopathy control program in Turkey. Public Health Genomics. 2006;**9**(2):124-126

[4] Weatherall DJ, Clegg JB. The Thalassaemia Syndromes. New York, NY: John Wiley and Sons; 2008

[5] Ribeil JA, Arlet JB, Dussiot M, Cruz Moura I, Courtois G, Hermine O. Ineffective erythropoiesis in β -thalassemia. Scientific World Journal. 2013;**2013**(1):394295

[6] Cao A, Galanello R. Beta-thalassemia. Genetics in Medicine. 2010;**12**(2):61-76

[7] Galanello R, Origa R. Beta-thalassemia. Orphanet Journal of Rare Diseases. 2010;**5**(1):11

[8] Sharma DC, Arya A, Kishor P, Woike P, Bindal J. Overview on thalassemias: A review article. Medico Research Chronicles. 2017;**4**(03):325-337

[9] Desforges JF, Eisenstein BI. The polymerase chain reaction: A new method of using molecular genetics for medical diagnosis. The New England Journal of Medicine. 1990;**322**(3):178-183

[10] Lindeman R, Hu SP, Volpato F, Trent RJ. Polymerase chain reaction (PCR) mutagenesis enabling rapid non-radioactive detection of common β-thalassaemia mutations in Mediterraneans. British Journal of Haematology. 1991;**78**(1):100-104

[11] Tan J. The use of amplification refractory mutation system (ARMS) as an effective and economical tool for prenatal diagnosis of β-thalassaemia in Malaysian subjects. Journal of International Medical Research. 1998;**2**:65-68

[12] Honardoost MA, Tabatabaeian H, Akbari M, Salehi M. Investigation of sensitivity, specificity and accuracy of tetra primer ARMS PCR method in comparison with conventional ARMS PCR, based on sequencing technique outcomes in IVS-II-I genotyping of beta thalassemia patients. Gene. 2014;**549**(1):1-6

[13] Agarwal S, Sarwai S, Nigam N, Singhal P. Rapid detection of ot thalassaemia deletion and o-globin gene triplication by gap-PCR in Indian subjects. The Indian Journal of Medical Research. 2002;**116**:155-161

[14] Tritipsombut J, Phylipsen M, Viprakasit V, Chalaow N, Sanchaisuriya K, Giordano PC, et al. A single-tube multiplex gap-polymerase chain reaction for the detection of eight β-globin gene cluster deletions common in Southeast Asia. Hemoglobin. 2012;**36**(6):571-580

[15] Moreno I, Bolufer P, Perez ML, Barragán E, Sanz MA. Rapid detection of the major Mediterranean β-thalassaemia mutations by real-time polymerase chain reaction using fluorophore-labelled hybridization probes. British Journal of Haematology. 2002;**119**(2):554-557

[16] Traeger-Synodinos J, Vrettou C, Kanavakis E. Rapid detection of fetal mendelian disorders: Thalassemia and sickle cell syndromes. In: Hahn S, Jackson LG, editors. Prenatal Diagnosis. Totowa, NJ: Humana Press; 2008. p. 133-145 (Walker JM, editor. Methods in Molecular Biology™; vol. 444) DOI: 10.1007/978-1-59745-066-9_10

[17] Seyed Jalal Marashi. Detection of eight common β-globin gene mutation in thalassemia major patients using real time polymerase chain reaction (PCR)-high resolution melting and EvaGreen™ dye. African Journal of Biotechnology. 2011;**11**(2):448

[18] Harteveld CL, Voskamp A, Phylipsen M, Akkermans N, den Dunnen JT, White SJ, et al. Nine unknown rearrangements in 16p13.3 and 11p15.4 causing α- and β-thalassaemia characterised by high resolution multiplex ligation-dependent probe amplification. Journal of Medical Genetics. 2005;**42**(12):922

[19] Onay H, Ekmekçi A, Ataman E, Akgül M, Vahabi A, Aydınok Y, et al. HBA mutations detected by MLPA in beta-thalassemia patients. European Journal of Therapeutics. 2009;**15**(1):1-4

[20] Phylipsen M, Prior JF, Lim E, Lingam N, Vogelaar IP, Giordano PC, et al. Thalassemia in Western Australia: 11 novel deletions characterized by multiplex ligation-dependent probe amplification. Blood Cells, Molecules and Diseases. 2010;**44**(3):146-151

[21] Cui J, Azimi M, Baysdorfer C, Vichinsky EP, Hoppe CC. Application of multiplex ligation-dependent probe amplification to screen for β-globin cluster deletions: Detection of two novel deletions in a multi ethnic population. Hemoglobin. 2013;**37**(3):241-256

[22] Joly P, Pondarre C, Badens C. Beta-thalassemias: Molecular, epidemiological, diagnostical and clinical aspects. Annales de biologie clinique. 2014;**72**(6):639-668

[23] Angastiniotis M, Eleftheriou A, Galanello R, Harteveld C, Petrou M, Traeger-Synodinos J, et al. Prevention of thalassaemias and other haemoglobin disorders: Volume 1: Principles. 2014

[24] Papasavva T, WFJ VI, CEM K, MCGN VDH, Kountouris P, Kythreotis L, et al. Next generation sequencing of SNPs for non-invasive prenatal diagnosis: Challenges and feasibility as illustrated by an application to β-thalassaemia. European Journal of Human Genetics. 2013;**21**(12):1403-1410

[25] Shooter C, Rooks H, Thein SL, Clark B. Next generation sequencing identifies a novel rearrangement in the *HBB* cluster permitting to-the-base characterization. Human Mutation. 2015;**36**(1):142-150

[26] He J, Song W, Yang J, Lu S, Yuan Y, Guo J, et al. Next-generation sequencing improves thalassemia carrier screening among premarital adults in a high prevalence population: The Dai nationality, China. Genetics in Medicine. 2017;**19**(9):1022-1031

[27] Phylipsen M, Yamsri S, Treffers EE, Jansen DTSL, Kanhai WA, Boon EMJ, et al. Non-invasive prenatal diagnosis of beta-thalassemia and sickle-cell disease using pyrophosphorolysis-activated polymerization and melting curve analysis. Prenatal Diagnosis. 2012;**32**(6):578-587

[28] Yenilmez ED, Tuli A, Evrüke İC. Noninvasive prenatal diagnosis experience in the Çukurova region of Southern Turkey: Detecting paternal mutations of sickle cell anemia and β-thalassemia in cell-free

fetal DNA using high-resolution melting analysis. Prenatal Diagnosis. 2013;**33**(11):1054-1062

[29] Prabhu R, Prabhu V, Prabhu R. Iron overload in beta thalassemia: A review. Journal of BioScience and Biotechnology. 2009;**1**(1):20-31

[30] Mishra AK, Tiwari A. Iron overload in beta thalassaemia major and intermedia patients. Maedica. 2013;**8**(4):328-332

[31] Musallam KM, Cappellini MD, Wood JC, Motta I, Graziadei G, Tamim H, et al. Elevated liver iron concentration is a marker of increased morbidity in patients with thalassemia intermedia. Haematologica. 2011;**96**(11):1605-1612

[32] Origa R, Galanello R, Ganz T, Giagu N, Maccioni L, Faa G, et al. Liver iron concentrations and urinary hepcidin in -thalassemia. Haematologica. 2007;**92**(5):583-588

[33] Pennell DJ. T2* magnetic resonance and myocardial iron in thalassemia. Annals of the New York Academy of Sciences. 2005;**1054**(1):373-378

[34] Kaltwasser J, Gottschalk R, Schalk K, Hartl W. Non-invasive quantitation of liver iron-overload by magnetic resonance imaging. British Journal of Haematology. 1990;**74**(3):360-363

[35] Chezmar JL, Nelson RC, Malko JA, Bernardino ME. Hepatic iron overload: Diagnosis and quantification by noninvasive imaging. Gastrointestinal Radiology. 1990;**15**:27-31

[36] De Sanctis V. Severe liver iron concentrations (Lic) In 24 patients with B-thalassemia major: Correlations with serum ferritin, liver enzymes and endocrine complications. Mediterranean Journal of Hematology and Infectious Diseases. 2018;**10**:e2018062

[37] Argyropoulou MI, Astrakas L. MRI evaluation of tissue iron burden in patients with β-thalassaemia major. Pediatric Radiology. 2007;**37**(12):1191-1200

[38] Christoforidis A, Haritandi A, Tsatra I, Tsitourides I, Karyda S, Athanassiou-Metaxa M. Four-year evaluation of myocardial and liver iron assessed prospectively with serial MRI scans in young patients with β-thalassaemia major: Comparison between different chelation regimens. European Journal of Haematology. 2007;**78**(1):52-57

[39] Md EA, Md TH, Md SM, Phd BB, Msc EL. Association between serum ferritin level, cardiac and hepatic T2-star MRI in patients with major β-thalassemia. Iranian journal of Pediatric Hematology and Oncology. 2014;**4**:17-21

[40] Hahalis G, Manolis AS, Apostolopoulos D, Alexopoulos D, Vagenakis AG, Zoumbos NC. Right ventricular cardiomyopathy in beta-thalassaemia major. European Heart Journal. 2002;**23**(2):147-156

[41] Aessopos A, Berdoukas VA. Mediterranean Journal of Hematology and Infectious Diseases Cardiac Function and Iron Chelation in Thalassemia Major and Intermedia: a Review of the Underlying Pathophysiology and Approach to Chelation Management. 2009. Available from: https://api.semanticscholar.org/CorpusID:11764496

[42] Russo V, Rago A, Papa AA, Nigro G. Electrocardiographic presentation, cardiac arrhythmias, and their management in β-thalassemia major

patients. Annals of Noninvasive Electrocardiology. 2016;**21**(4):335-342

[43] Carpenter JP, Roughton M, Pennell DJ. The myocardial iron in thalassemia (MINT) investigators. International survey of T2* cardiovascular magnetic resonance in -thalassemia major. Haematologica. 2013;**98**(9):1368-1374

[44] Aldouri MA, Wonke B, Hoffbrand AV, Flynn DM, Ward SE, Agnew JE, et al. High incidence of cardiomyopathy in Beta-thalassaemia patients receiving regular transfusion and iron chelation: Reversal by intensified chelation. Acta Haematologica. 1990;**84**(3):113-117

[45] Chaosuwannakit N, Makarawate P, Wanitpongpun C. The importance of cardiac T2* magnetic resonance imaging for monitoring cardiac siderosis in thalassemia major patients. Tomography. 2021;**7**(2):130-138

[46] Aydinok Y. Endocrine complications in patients with -thalassemia major. Journal of Tropical Pediatrics. 2002;**48**(1):50-54

[47] Najafipour F, Aliasgarzadeh A, Aghamohamadzadeh N, Bahrami A, Mobasri M, Niafar M, et al. A cross-sectional study of metabolic and endocrine complications in beta-thalassemia major. Annals of Saudi Medicine. 2008;**28**(5):361-366

[48] Malik SA, Syed S, Ahmed N. Frequency of hypothyroidism in patients of beta-thalassaemia. JPMA. Journal of the Pakistan Medical Association. 2010;**60**(1):17-20

[49] El-Hazmi MAF, Warsy AS, Al-Fawaz I. Iron-endocrine pattern in patients with -thalassaemia. Journal of Tropical Pediatrics. 1994;**40**(4):219-224

[50] Hagag AA, Badraia IM, Elfarargy MS, Abo El-Enein AM. Gonadal hormones in adolescent females with β-thalassemia in relation to iron load. Endocrine, Metabolic and Immune Disorders—Drug Targets. 2016;**16**(2):148-153

[51] Gullo L, Corcioni E, Brancati C, Bria M, Pezzilli R, Sprovieri G. Morphologic and functional evaluation of the exocrine pancreas in β-thalassemia major. Pancreas. 1993;**8**(2):176-180

[52] Midiri M, Lo Casto A, Sparacia G, D'Angelo P, Malizia R, Finazzo M, et al. MR imaging of pancreatic changes in patients with transfusion-dependent beta-thalassemia major. American Journal of Roentgenology. 1999;**173**(1):187-192

[53] Noetzli LJ, Mittelman SD, Watanabe RM, Coates TD, Wood JC. Pancreatic iron and glucose dysregulation in thalassemia major. American Journal of Hematology. 2012;**87**(2):155-160

[54] Dundar U, Kupesiz A, Ozdem S, Gilgil E, Tuncer T, Yeşilipek A, et al. Bone metabolism and mineral density in patients with beta-thalassemia major. Saudi Medical Journal. 2007;**28**(9):1425-1429

[55] Perisano C, Marzetti E, Spinelli MS, Callà CAM, Graci C, Maccauro G. Physiopathology of bone modifications in β -thalassemia. Anemia. 2012;**2012**:1-5

[56] Haidar R, Musallam KM, Taher AT. Bone disease and skeletal complications in patients with β thalassemia major. Bone. 2011;**48**(3):425-432

[57] Pollak RD, Rachmilewitz E, Blumenfeld A, Idelson M, Goldfarb AW. Bone mineral metabolism in adults with beta-thalassaemia major and intermedia.

British Journal of Haematology. 2000;**111**(3):902-907

[58] Barry M, Flynn DM, Letsky EA, Risdon RA. Long-term chelation therapy in thalassaemia major: Effect on liver iron concentration, liver histology, and clinical progress. BMJ. 1974;**2**(5909):16-20

[59] Chelation Therapy [Internet]. Northern California Comprehensive Thalassemia Center. 2024. Available from: https://thalassemia.ucsf.edu/chelation-therapy

[60] Gandon Y, Olivie D, Guyader D, Aubé C, Oberti F, Sebille V, et al. Non-invasive assessment of hepatic iron stores by MRI. The Lancet. 2004;**363**(9406):357-362

[61] Guzelbey T, Gurses B, Ozturk E, Ozveren O, Sarsilmaz A, Karasu E. Evaluation of iron deposition in the adrenal glands of β thalassemia major patients using 3-tesla MRI. Iranian Journal of Radiology. 10 May 2016;**13**(3):e36375

[62] Guzelbey T, Demirbaş ZE, Gurses B. The Evaluation of Renal Iron Deposition With a 3 Tesla MRI Device in Beta-Thalassemia Major Patients. Cureus. Mar 2023;**15**(3):e36179

[63] Guo H, Au W, Cheung JS, Kim D, Jensen JH, Khong P, et al. Myocardial T2 quantitation in patients with iron overload at 3 tesla. Journal of Magnetic Resonance Imaging. 2009;**30**(2):394-400

[64] Nayak AM, Choudhari A, Patkar DP, Merchant RH. Pituitary volume and iron overload evaluation by 3T MRI in thalassemia. Indian Journal of Pediatrics. 2021;**88**:656-662

[65] Qiu D, Chan GF, Chu J, Chan Q, Ha SY, Moseley M, et al. MR quantitative susceptibility imaging for the evaluation of iron loading in the brains of patients with β-thalassemia major. American Journal of Neuroradiology. 2014;**35**(6):1085-1090

[66] Lun FM, Tsui NB, Chan KA, Leung TY, Lau TK, Charoenkwan P, et al. Noninvasive prenatal diagnosis of monogenic diseases by digital size selection and relative mutation dosage on DNA in maternal plasma. Proceedings of the National Academy of Sciences. 2008;**105**(50):19920-19925

[67] Zafari M, Kosaryan M, Gill P, Alipour A, Shiran M, Jalalli H, et al. Non-invasive prenatal diagnosis of β-thalassemia by detection of the cell-free fetal DNA in maternal circulation: A systematic review and meta-analysis. Annals of Hematology. 2016;**95**(8):1341-1350

[68] Jayashankar SS, Nasaruddin ML, Hassan MF, Dasrilsyah RA, Shafiee MN, Ismail NAS, et al. Non-invasive prenatal testing (NIPT): Reliability, challenges, and future directions. Diagnostics. 2023;**13**(15):2570

[69] Mousavi S, Shokri Z, Bastani P, Ghojazadeh M, Riahifar S, Nateghian H. Factors affecting low fetal fraction in fetal screening with cell-free DNA in pregnant women: A systematic review and meta-analysis. BMC Pregnancy and Childbirth. 2022;**22**(1):918

[70] Xiong L, Barrett AN, Hua R, Tan TZ, Ho SSY, Chan JK, et al. Non-invasive prenatal diagnostic testing for β-thalassaemia using cell-free fetal DNA and next generation sequencing. Prenatal Diagnosis. 2015;**35**(3):258-265

[71] Sabiha B, Haider SA, Jan H, Yousafzai YM, Afridi OK, Khan AA, et al. Development of the next generation sequencing-based diagnostic test for β-thalassemia and its validation

in a Pashtun family. Hemoglobin. 2020;**44**(4):254-258

[72] Yin ZZ, Yao J, Wei FX, Chen CY, Yan HM, Zhang M. Targeted next-generation sequencing reveals a large novel β-thalassemia deletion that removes the entire *HBB* gene. Hemoglobin. 2022;**46**(5):290-295

[73] Erlich HA, López-Peña C, Carlberg KT, Shih S, Bali G, Yamaguchi KD, et al. Noninvasive prenatal test for β-thalassemia and sickle cell disease using probe capture enrichment and next-generation sequencing of DNA in maternal plasma. Journal of Applied Laboratory Medicine. 2022;**7**(2):515-531

[74] Liang Q, Gu W, Chen P, Li Y, Liu Y, Tian M, et al. A more universal approach to comprehensive analysis of thalassemia alleles (CATSA). The Journal of Molecular Diagnostics. 2021;**23**(9):1195-1204

[75] Zhan L, Gui C, Wei W, Liu J, Gui B. Third generation sequencing transforms the way of the screening and diagnosis of thalassemia: A mini-review. Frontiers in Pediatrics. 2023;**11**:1199609

[76] Xu Z, Hu L, Liu Y, Peng C, Zeng G, Zeng L, et al. Comparison of third-generation sequencing and routine polymerase chain reaction in genetic analysis of thalassemia. Archives of Pathology and Laboratory Medicine. 2024;**148**(3):336-344

[77] Risoluti R, Materazzi S, Sorrentino F, Maffei L, Caprari P. Thermogravimetric analysis coupled with chemometrics as a powerful predictive tool for ß-thalassemia screening. Talanta. 2016;**159**:425-432

[78] Risoluti R, Materazzi S, Sorrentino F, Bozzi C, Caprari P. Update on thalassemia diagnosis: New insights and methods. Talanta. 2018;**183**:216-222

[79] Ferih K, Elsayed B, Elshoeibi AM, Elsabagh AA, Elhadary M, Soliman A, et al. Applications of artificial intelligence in thalassemia: A comprehensive review. Diagnostics. 2023;**13**(9):1551

[80] Abdulkarim D, Abdulazeez AM. Machine learning-based prediction of thalassemia: A review. Indonesian Journal of Electrical Engineering and Computer Science. 15 Jun 2024;**13**(3):4046-4071

[81] Wongseree W, Chaiyaratana N, Vichittumaros K, Winichagoon P, Fucharoen S. Thalassaemia classification by neural networks and genetic programming. Information Sciences. 2007;**177**(3):771-786

[82] Barnhart-Magen G, Gotlib V, Marilus R, Einav Y. Differential diagnostics of thalassemia minor by artificial neural networks model. Journal of Clinical Laboratory Analysis. 2013;**27**(6):481-486

[83] Kaur G, Garg VK. A systematic review on thalassemia using neural network techniques. ACM Journal on Emerging Technologies in Computing Systems. 2024:519-524

[84] Shen C, Jiang YM, Shi H, Hao LJ, Jie ZW, Kai DQ, et al. Evaluation of indices in differentiation between iron deficiency anemia and β-thalassemia trait for Chinese children. Journal of Pediatric Hematology/Oncology. 2010;**32**(6):e218-e222

[85] Kabootarizadeh L, Jamshidnezhad A, Koohmareh Z, Ghamchili A. Differential diagnosis of iron-deficiency anemia from beta-thalassemia trait using an intelligent model in comparison with discriminant

indexes. Acta Informatica Medica. 2019;**27**(2):78

[86] Matos JF, Dusse LMS, Borges KBG, De Castro RLV, Coura-Vital W, Carvalho MDG. A new index to discriminate between iron deficiency anemia and thalassemia trait. Revista Brasileira de Hematologia e Hemoterapia. 2016;**38**(3):214-219

[87] Laengsri V, Shoombuatong W, Adirojananon W, Nantasenamat C, Prachayasittikul V, Nuchnoi P. ThalPred: A web-based prediction tool for discriminating thalassemia trait and iron deficiency anemia. BMC Medical Informatics and Decision Making. 2019;**19**:1-14

[88] Positano V, Meloni A, Santarelli MF, Pistoia L, Spasiano A, Cuccia L, et al. Deep learning staging of liver iron content from multiecho MR images. Journal of Magnetic Resonance Imaging. 2023;**57**(2):472-484

[89] Asmarian N, Kamalipour A, Hosseini-Bensenjan M, Karimi M, Haghpanah S. Prediction of heart and liver iron overload in β-thalassemia major patients using machine learning methods. Hemoglobin. 2022;**46**(6):303-307

[90] Taleie H, Hajianfar G, Sabouri M, Parsaee M, Houshmand G, Bitarafan-Rajabi A, et al. Left ventricular myocardial dysfunction evaluation in thalassemia patients using echocardiographic radiomic features and machine learning algorithms. Journal of Digital Imaging. 2023;**36**(6):2494-2506

[91] Yousefian F, Banirostam T, Azarkeivan A. Predicting the risk of diabetes in Iranian patients with β-thalassemia major/intermedia based on artificial neural network. Signal Process Renew Energy. 2019;**3**(4):23-33

[92] Agarwal RK, Sedai A, Ankita K, Parmar L, Dhanya R, Dhimal S, et al. Information technology–assisted treatment planning and performance assessment for severe thalassemia care in low-and middle-income countries: Observational study. JMIR Medical Informatics. 2019;**7**(1):e9291

[93] Santini S, Pescapè A, Valente AS, Abate V, Improta G, Triassi M, et al. Using Fuzzy Logic for Improving Clinical Daily-Care of β-Thalassemia Patients. Naples: IEEE; 2017. pp. 1-6

[94] Tran DC, Dang AL, Hoang TNL, Nguyen CT, Le TMP, Dinh TNM, et al. Prevalence of thalassemia in the Vietnamese population and building a clinical decision support system for prenatal screening for thalassemia. Mediterranean Journal of Hematology and Infectious Diseases. 2023;**15**(1):e2023026

Chapter 5

Nutritional Therapy: A Complementary Approach in the Management of Inherited Blood Disorders

Mahdi Karimi

Abstract

Nutritional therapy is increasingly recognized as a vital component in managing inherited blood disorders. This chapter explores the role of tailored nutritional interventions in addressing the specific needs of patients with conditions such as thalassemia and sickle cell disease. Key areas include adjusting energy, protein, fat, and carbohydrate intake, and supplementing with micronutrients like iron, folic acid, and vitamin D. The chapter also examines dietary interventions, the integration of nutrition with conventional treatments, and challenges such as compliance and cultural factors. Emerging research in nutrigenomics and advanced supplements promises personalized and effective therapies. The future of nutritional therapy lies in its integration into standard care practices, guided by evidence-based research and a multidisciplinary approach. This holistic strategy aims to enhance patient outcomes and improve the quality of life for individuals with inherited blood disorders.

Keywords: nutritional therapy, inherited blood disorders, micronutrient supplementation, personalized nutrition, dietary interventions

1. Introduction

Inherited blood disorders, such as thalassemia, sickle cell disease, and hemophilia, represent a significant global health burden affecting millions of individuals worldwide. These disorders are characterized by genetic mutations that result in abnormal production or function of blood cells, leading to a range of clinical complications. Traditional management of these conditions has primarily focused on pharmacological interventions, including blood transfusions, chelation therapy, and, in some cases, bone marrow transplantation. However, despite advances in medical treatment, managing inherited blood disorders remains complex and often requires a multidisciplinary approach.

Nutritional therapy has emerged as a complementary strategy in the management of inherited blood disorders, offering potential benefits in improving patient outcomes and quality of life. Nutritional status is closely linked to the pathophysiology of these disorders, with deficiencies in specific micronutrients contributing to disease progression and complications. For instance, iron overload in patients with thalassemia necessitates careful monitoring and dietary management, while individuals with sickle cell disease may benefit from antioxidant-rich diets to mitigate oxidative stress.

This chapter aims to explore the role of nutritional therapy in the management of inherited blood disorders, highlighting its potential as an adjunct to conventional treatments. We will examine the specific nutritional needs of patients with these conditions, the impact of micronutrient supplementation, and the potential for dietary interventions to improve clinical outcomes. Additionally, the chapter will address the challenges associated with implementing nutritional therapy in this patient population, including issues related to compliance, cultural factors, and the need for personalized approaches.

Through a comprehensive review of current research and clinical practice, this chapter seeks to provide healthcare professionals with practical insights into the integration of nutritional therapy into the standard care of patients with inherited blood disorders. By doing so, we hope to underscore the importance of a holistic approach to patient management that considers not only the pharmacological but also the nutritional aspects of care.

2. Nutritional requirements in inherited blood disorders

Nutritional status plays a critical role in the overall health and well-being of individuals with inherited blood disorders. These conditions often lead to specific nutritional deficiencies or imbalances that can exacerbate disease progression and impact the patient's quality of life. Understanding the unique nutritional requirements of these patients is essential for optimizing their care and supporting long-term health outcomes.

2.1 General nutritional needs

Patients with inherited blood disorders require a well-balanced diet that provides adequate energy, macronutrients, and micronutrients to support their physiological needs. Due to the chronic nature of these conditions, there is often an increased demand for certain nutrients to compensate for ongoing metabolic stress and complications associated with the disease. Key considerations include:

2.1.1 Energy requirements

2.1.1.1 Thalassemia

Energy needs for patients with thalassemia are typically 120–130% of the recommended daily allowance (RDA) for their age and sex due to increased metabolic demands [1]. For example, a 10-year-old child with thalassemia might require 1800 to 2100 kcal/day compared to the standard 1500 kcal/day.

2.1.1.2 Sickle cell disease

Patients with sickle cell disease also have increased energy needs, ranging from 120–150% of the RDA, particularly during periods of growth or infection [2]. An adolescent with sickle cell disease may require 2700 to 3000 kcal/day compared to the standard 2000 kcal/day for their age.

2.1.2 Protein intake

2.1.2.1 Thalassemia

Patients typically require 1.2 to 1.5 g/kg/day of protein to support muscle maintenance and recovery [3]. For a 50 kg adult, this translates to 60 to 75 g of protein per day.

2.1.2.2 Sickle cell disease

Protein requirements are also elevated, ranging from 1.5 to 2 g/kg/day to compensate for the increased turnover of red blood cells and to support growth and tissue repair [4]. For a 30 kg child, this would amount to 45 to 60 g of protein per day.

2.1.3 Fat and carbohydrate balance

2.1.3.1 General considerations

A balanced diet should include 20–35% of total energy intake from fats and 45–65% from carbohydrates, tailored to the patient's needs [5].

2.1.3.2 Thalassemia

Given the risk of NAFLD in thalassemia patients, it's recommended to limit saturated fat to less than 7% of total calories and to emphasize the intake of monounsaturated and polyunsaturated fats, particularly omega-3 fatty acids [6]. This equates to about 35–50 g of total fat per day for an adult consuming 2000 kcal/day, with less than 14 g of saturated fat.

2.1.3.3 Sickle cell disease

A diet rich in complex carbohydrates, high in fiber, and low in simple sugars is advisable. Carbohydrates should constitute 50–60% of the total energy intake, focusing on whole grains, fruits, and vegetables [7].

The following **Table 1** presents an overview of the recommended nutritional requirements specifically tailored for individuals with inherited blood disorders, including thalassemia and sickle cell disease. These guidelines reflect the unique metabolic demands and nutrient needs associated with these conditions.

Nutrient	Thalassemia	Sickle cell disease	References
Energy (kcal/day)	30–40 kcal/kg body weight, higher during periods of illness.	20–30% above normal energy needs due to increased metabolism.	[8, 9]
Protein (g/day)	1.2–1.5 g/kg body weight.	1.5–2.0 g/kg body weight, higher during crisis.	[9, 10]
Fat (% of total kcal)	25–35% of total caloric intake.	30–35% of total caloric intake.	[8, 11]
Carbohydrates (% of total kcal)	45–65% of total caloric intake.	50–60% of total caloric intake.	[8, 9]

Table 1.
Overview of recommended nutritional requirements for individuals with inherited blood disorders, including conditions like thalassemia and sickle cell disease.

2.1.4 Notes

2.1.4.1 Thalassemia

Patients often require lower iron intake due to the risk of iron overload, especially in those undergoing frequent transfusions. Calcium and vitamin D intake are crucial to mitigate the risk of osteoporosis.

2.1.4.2 Sickle cell disease

Increased energy and protein needs are due to hypermetabolism and the body's increased demand during vaso-occlusive crises. Zinc and folic acid are essential for managing anemia and immune function.

3. Micronutrient supplementation

Micronutrient supplementation is crucial in managing inherited blood disorders, given the increased risk of deficiencies due to the chronic nature of these diseases, frequent medical treatments, and specific disease-related metabolic demands. The following subsections address the critical micronutrients that require careful management in these patients.

3.1 Iron and iron-chelation therapy

3.1.1 Iron overload in thalassemia

Patients with thalassemia, particularly those who are transfusion-dependent, are at high risk for iron overload due to the regular transfusions they receive. Iron overload can lead to severe complications such as liver cirrhosis, cardiac dysfunction, and endocrine abnormalities.

3.1.1.1 Iron-chelation therapy

To manage iron overload, chelation therapy is essential. Deferoxamine, deferasirox, and deferiprone are commonly used iron chelators. The dosing for deferasirox is typically 20–40 mg/kg/day, depending on the degree of iron overload, to maintain serum ferritin levels below 1000 ng/mL [12].

3.1.1.2 Monitoring

Regular monitoring of serum ferritin and liver iron concentration using MRI is recommended to adjust chelation therapy accordingly [13].

3.1.2 Iron deficiency in non-transfusion-dependent thalassemia and sickle cell disease

While iron overload is a concern in transfusion-dependent patients, iron deficiency can occur in those who are non-transfusion-dependent. In such cases, iron supplementation should be administered cautiously to avoid exacerbating the risk of overload.

3.1.2.1 Supplementation

When necessary, oral iron supplementation should be given at doses of 60–120 mg of elemental iron per day [14], along with regular monitoring of iron status.

3.2 Role of folic acid and vitamin B12

3.2.1 Folic acid

Folic acid is essential for DNA synthesis and red blood cell production. Patients with inherited blood disorders, especially those undergoing regular hemolysis, such as in sickle cell disease and thalassemia, have increased folate requirements.

3.2.1.1 Supplementation

It is recommended that these patients take 1 mg of folic acid daily to prevent megaloblastic anemia and support erythropoiesis [15].

3.2.2 Vitamin B12

Vitamin B12 is crucial for maintaining healthy nerve cells and aiding in the production of DNA and red blood cells. Deficiency in vitamin B12 can lead to pernicious anemia and neurological complications.

3.2.2.1 Supplementation

Patients with vitamin B12 deficiency should receive 1000 mcg of vitamin B12 (cobalamin) daily, either orally or via intramuscular injections, depending on the severity of the deficiency [16].

3.3 Vitamin D and bone health

3.3.1 Bone disease in thalassemia

Thalassemia patients are at high risk of developing bone diseases such as osteoporosis and osteopenia due to both iron overload and the effects of iron-chelation therapy. Vitamin D plays a vital role in calcium homeostasis and bone mineralization.

3.3.1.1 Supplementation

To maintain bone health, a daily intake of 1000–2000 IU of vitamin D is recommended, with higher doses potentially necessary in cases of deficiency [17]. Calcium supplementation should also be considered, with a daily intake of 1000–1500 mg, depending on dietary intake and serum calcium levels [18].

3.3.2 Bone health in sickle cell disease

Patients with sickle cell disease also face a heightened risk of bone complications, including avascular necrosis and osteoporosis, partly due to chronic inflammation and reduced physical activity.

3.3.2.1 Supplementation

Similar to thalassemia patients, those with sickle cell disease should receive 1000–2000 IU of vitamin D daily, adjusted based on serum levels and seasonal exposure to sunlight [1].

3.4 Antioxidants and oxidative stress management

3.4.1 Oxidative stress in sickle cell disease

Oxidative stress plays a significant role in the pathophysiology of sickle cell disease, contributing to hemolysis and vaso-occlusive crises. Antioxidants can help mitigate oxidative damage and improve clinical outcomes.

3.4.1.1 Vitamin E

As a potent antioxidant, vitamin E supplementation at 400 IU/day is recommended to reduce oxidative stress and hemolysis in patients with sickle cell disease [2].

3.4.1.2 Vitamin C

Vitamin C also helps combat oxidative stress by regenerating other antioxidants. A dose of 500 mg/day is suggested, with caution to avoid excessive intake that might enhance iron absorption in patients at risk of iron overload [3].

3.4.1.3 Other antioxidants

Additional antioxidants like selenium (50–100 mcg/day) and zinc (30–50 mg/day) can also support oxidative stress management and improve immune function in these patients [4].

provides a comprehensive summary of the micronutrient supplementation requirements for individuals with inherited blood disorders, such as thalassemia and sickle cell disease. **Table 2** outlines the recommended dosages for various essential micronutrients, highlighting their role in managing the specific challenges associated with these conditions.

3.5 Notes

3.5.1 Thalassemia

Iron supplementation is generally avoided due to the risk of iron overload, particularly in patients receiving regular blood transfusions. The focus is on other micronutrients to support bone health and prevent anemia.

3.5.2 Sickle cell disease

Nutrient supplementation aims to support the immune system, manage anemia, and reduce oxidative stress. Regular monitoring is essential to adjust dosages based on individual needs.

Micronutrient	Thalassemia	Sickle cell disease	References
Iron	Avoid supplementation; use iron-chelation therapy as needed.	Avoid supplementation; monitor for overload.	[5, 6]
Folic acid (μg/day)	800–1000 μg/day, particularly important for managing anemia.	1000 μg/day, especially during periods of increased hemolysis.	[7, 12]
Vitamin B12 (μg/day)	2.4–6 μg/day depending on deficiency status.	3–6 μg/day, may require higher doses in case of deficiency.	[5, 13]
Vitamin D (IU/day)	600–1000 IU/day, higher if deficiency or osteoporosis present.	800–1000 IU/day, monitor levels regularly.	[13, 17]
Calcium (mg/day)	1000–1300 mg/day, particularly important due to risk of osteoporosis.	1000–1300 mg/day, combined with vitamin D supplementation.	[5, 13]
Zinc (mg/day)	8–11 mg/day can help improve immune function and reduce oxidative stress.	10–15 mg/day, beneficial for wound healing and immune support.	[7, 19]
Selenium (μg/day)	55–75 μg/day may help reduce oxidative stress.	55–75 μg/day, potential role in reducing hemolysis.	[5, 19]
Vitamin E (mg/day)	15–30 mg/day, antioxidant to reduce oxidative damage.	15–30 mg/day, supports immune function and reduces hemolysis.	[13, 19]

Table 2.
Summary of recommended dosages for key micronutrient supplements in managing inherited blood disorders.

4. Dietary interventions

Dietary interventions are a cornerstone of managing inherited blood disorders, as they can significantly impact disease progression, symptom management, and overall quality of life. This section explores the importance of diet plans tailored to specific disorders, the role of functional foods, and the broader impact of diet on patients' well-being.

4.1 Diet plans tailored to specific disorders

Each inherited blood disorder presents unique nutritional challenges, necessitating tailored diet plans to address specific needs:

4.1.1 Thalassemia

4.1.1.1 Iron management

Given the risk of iron overload, it is critical to limit dietary iron intake in thalassemia patients, particularly those who are transfusion-dependent. Red meats and iron-fortified foods should be minimized, while foods high in calcium and polyphenols (e.g., tea and coffee) that inhibit iron absorption can be included strategically [20].

4.1.1.2 Balanced nutrition

A well-rounded diet rich in fruits, vegetables, and whole grains is recommended to provide essential nutrients while avoiding excess iron. Patients should also focus on foods that support bone health, such as dairy products and leafy greens, to mitigate the risk of osteoporosis [21].

4.1.2 Sickle cell disease

4.1.2.1 Hydration and caloric intake

Adequate hydration is vital in sickle cell disease to prevent sickling crises. Patients should consume at least 8–10 glasses of water daily, with higher intake during hot weather or physical activity [14]. Caloric needs are elevated, especially during periods of increased metabolic stress, such as infection or vaso-occlusive episodes. A diet rich in complex carbohydrates, lean proteins, and healthy fats is recommended to meet these increased energy demands [16].

4.1.2.2 Anti-inflammatory diet

Incorporating anti-inflammatory foods like fatty fish (rich in omega-3 fatty acids), nuts, and seeds can help manage chronic inflammation associated with sickle cell disease [22].

4.2 Role of functional foods

Functional foods—those that offer health benefits beyond basic nutrition—can play a significant role in managing inherited blood disorders.

4.2.1 Probiotics and gut health

The gut microbiome's role in inflammation and immunity has led to growing interest in probiotics for patients with inherited blood disorders. Probiotic-rich foods such as yogurt, kefir, and fermented vegetables can support gut health and potentially reduce inflammation in conditions like sickle cell disease [8].

4.2.2 Antioxidant-rich foods

Foods high in antioxidants, such as berries, dark chocolate, and green tea, can help mitigate oxidative stress, a common challenge in both thalassemia and sickle cell disease. Regular consumption of these foods may reduce the frequency of oxidative damage and improve overall health outcomes [9].

4.2.3 Omega-3 fatty acids

Omega-3 fatty acids, found in fatty fish (like salmon and mackerel), flaxseeds, and walnuts, have anti-inflammatory properties. Incorporating these into the diet can be particularly beneficial for managing inflammation and reducing the risk of complications in sickle cell disease [11].

4.3 Impact of diet on quality of life

Dietary management is not just about addressing clinical symptoms; it also plays a crucial role in enhancing the overall quality of life for individuals with inherited blood disorders.

4.3.1 Physical well-being

A well-balanced diet can help reduce the frequency of disease-related complications, leading to fewer hospitalizations and a better physical state. For example, adequate hydration and a nutrient-rich diet can prevent vaso-occlusive crises in sickle cell patients, allowing for more consistent participation in daily activities [23].

4.3.2 Mental health

Nutritional status is closely linked to mental health. Deficiencies in essential nutrients like omega-3 fatty acids, B vitamins, and minerals can contribute to mood disorders, including depression and anxiety. A diet that supports mental well-being can enhance patients' ability to cope with the psychological burden of chronic illness [10].

4.3.3 Social and emotional well-being

Dietary restrictions and the need for specialized diets can impact social interactions and emotional well-being. Providing patients with flexible, enjoyable diet plans that allow them to participate in social activities without feeling restricted can significantly improve their quality of life [24].

5. Interaction of nutrition with conventional treatments

Nutritional therapy can play a significant role alongside conventional pharmacological treatments in managing inherited blood disorders. This section explores how nutritional interventions can act as adjuvants to traditional therapies, discusses the potential benefits and risks, and provides case studies and clinical evidence supporting these approaches.

5.1 Nutritional therapy as an adjuvant to pharmacological treatments

Nutritional interventions can complement pharmacological treatments by enhancing their efficacy, reducing side effects, and improving overall patient outcomes.

5.1.1 Thalassemia

5.1.1.1 Chelation therapy

In patients with thalassemia undergoing iron-chelation therapy, the inclusion of specific nutrients can enhance the effectiveness of treatment. For instance, ascorbic acid (vitamin C) at low doses (50–100 mg/day) can increase the excretion of iron when taken alongside chelators like deferoxamine [25]. However, excessive vitamin C can exacerbate iron overload, highlighting the need for careful monitoring [12].

5.1.1.2 Bone health

Nutritional support with calcium and vitamin D can help mitigate the bone density loss often associated with long-term chelation therapy. Patients receiving bisphosphonates for osteoporosis may benefit from increased dietary calcium (1000–1500 mg/day) and vitamin D (1,000–2000 IU/day) to optimize treatment outcomes [13].

5.1.2 Sickle cell disease

5.1.2.1 Hydroxyurea therapy

Hydroxyurea, a common treatment for sickle cell disease, increases fetal hemoglobin levels, reducing the frequency of vaso-occlusive crises. Adequate folate intake (1 mg/day) is essential for patients on hydroxyurea to support increased red blood cell production and prevent anemia [14]. Additionally, antioxidants such as vitamin E (400 IU/day) may reduce the oxidative stress associated with hydroxyurea therapy, potentially enhancing its therapeutic effects [15].

5.1.2.2 Pain management

Omega-3 fatty acids, found in fish oil supplements, have shown promise in reducing the frequency and severity of pain episodes in sickle cell disease when used alongside conventional pain management strategies. Doses of 1–2 grams/day of EPA and DHA combined have been suggested for their anti-inflammatory effects [16].

5.2 Potential benefits and risks

While nutritional therapy offers significant benefits as an adjunct to conventional treatments, it also carries potential risks that must be carefully managed.

5.2.1 Benefits

5.2.1.1 Enhanced efficacy of treatments

Nutritional support can improve the efficacy of pharmacological treatments by providing the necessary substrates for metabolic processes, reducing side effects, and addressing comorbid conditions. For example, vitamin D supplementation has been shown to enhance the response to bisphosphonate therapy in thalassemia patients with osteoporosis [17].

5.2.1.2 Improved quality of life

By addressing nutritional deficiencies, patients may experience improved energy levels, reduced symptoms, and a better overall quality of life. For instance, zinc supplementation in sickle cell disease has been linked to fewer sickle cell crises and improved immune function [26].

5.2.2 Risks

5.2.2.1 Nutrient-treatment interactions

Certain nutrients can interact with medications, either enhancing or inhibiting their effects. For instance, high doses of vitamin C can increase iron absorption, potentially worsening iron overload in thalassemia patients [19]. Similarly, excessive vitamin K intake may interfere with anticoagulant therapy, posing a risk for patients with thrombotic complications [21].

5.2.2.2 Over-supplementation

The risk of over-supplementation is a concern, particularly in patients already receiving multiple medications. Excessive intake of fat-soluble vitamins (A, D, E, and K) can lead to toxicity, while high doses of minerals like iron or zinc may disrupt the balance of other essential nutrients [24].

5.3 Case studies and clinical evidence

Clinical evidence supporting the role of nutrition in conjunction with conventional treatments is growing, with several case studies and trials demonstrating positive outcomes:

5.3.1 Case study: Omega-3 fatty acids in sickle cell disease

A study involving sickle cell disease patients supplemented with omega-3 fatty acids (1.2 grams of EPA and 0.9 grams of DHA daily) showed a significant reduction in the frequency of vaso-occlusive crises and improved overall well-being over 12 months [23]. These findings suggest that omega-3 supplementation may serve as a valuable adjunct to standard care in managing sickle cell disease.

5.3.2 Clinical trial: Vitamin D and bone health in thalassemia

A randomized controlled trial in patients with thalassemia major demonstrated that vitamin D supplementation (2000 IU/day) significantly improved bone mineral density and reduced the risk of fractures when combined with standard bisphosphonate therapy [8]. This trial underscores the importance of addressing vitamin D deficiency to optimize bone health in these patients.

5.3.3 Observational study: Antioxidants and hydroxyurea therapy

An observational study in patients with sickle cell disease receiving hydroxyurea found that those who also took antioxidants (vitamins C and E) had fewer hospitalizations for pain crises and better overall clinical outcomes [25]. These results highlight the potential for antioxidants to enhance the therapeutic effects of hydroxyurea.

6. Challenges and considerations in nutritional therapy

Nutritional therapy for inherited blood disorders involves several challenges and considerations that can impact the effectiveness of treatment and patient adherence. This section addresses key issues such as compliance and cultural factors, managing side effects, and the importance of nutritional assessment and monitoring.

6.1 Compliance and cultural factors

6.1.1 Patient adherence

6.1.1.1 Complex regimens

Adhering to dietary recommendations can be challenging due to the complexity of regimens, particularly when multiple supplements or dietary restrictions are involved. Patients may struggle with maintaining a consistent intake of specific nutrients or avoiding certain foods [24].

6.1.1.2 Education and support

Providing comprehensive education about the importance of dietary interventions and involving patients in the development of their dietary plans can improve adherence. Regular follow-up and support from dietitians can also enhance patient compliance [10].

6.1.2 Cultural considerations

6.1.2.1 Dietary preferences

Cultural dietary practices and food preferences can significantly influence adherence to nutritional recommendations. Tailoring dietary plans to accommodate cultural preferences while still meeting therapeutic goals is crucial for effective management [27].

6.1.2.2 Social and economic factors

Socioeconomic status can affect access to certain foods and supplements. Ensuring that dietary recommendations are feasible within the patient's economic and social context helps in achieving better compliance [11].

6.2 Managing side effects

6.2.1 Supplement interactions

6.2.1.1 Potential interactions

Nutritional supplements can interact with medications, potentially affecting their efficacy or causing adverse effects. For example, excessive vitamin C intake can increase iron absorption, which may be problematic for patients with thalassemia [9]. Monitoring and adjusting supplement doses based on individual needs is essential to avoid adverse interactions.

6.2.1.2 Adverse reactions

Some supplements may cause gastrointestinal distress or allergic reactions. Patients should be monitored for any adverse reactions, and alternative options should be considered if side effects occur [27].

6.2.2 Balancing nutrient intake

6.2.2.1 Over-supplementation risks

Over-supplementation of certain nutrients, such as fat-soluble vitamins (A, D, E, and K), can lead to toxicity. Regular assessment of nutrient levels and careful management of supplementation doses are necessary to avoid such risks [28].

6.2.2.2 Nutrient imbalances

Maintaining a balanced intake of nutrients is important to prevent imbalances that could affect overall health. For example, high doses of zinc can interfere with copper absorption, leading to deficiencies [29].

6.3 Nutritional assessment and monitoring

6.3.1 Regular monitoring

6.3.1.1 Nutrient status

Regular assessment of nutrient levels through blood tests and other diagnostic measures helps ensure that patients are meeting their nutritional needs and allows for timely adjustments to their dietary plans [30]. For instance, monitoring iron levels in thalassemia patients is critical to adjust chelation therapy and avoid iron overload [31].

6.3.1.2 Clinical outcomes

Tracking clinical outcomes such as bone mineral density, growth parameters, and frequency of disease-related events provides valuable feedback on the effectiveness of nutritional interventions [32].

6.3.2 Personalized plans

6.3.2.1 Individual needs

Nutritional therapy should be personalized based on individual health status, disease severity, and response to treatment. Regular reviews and adjustments of dietary plans ensure that they remain aligned with the patient's evolving needs and treatment goals [33].

6.3.2.2 Integration with other therapies

Coordination with other healthcare providers, including physicians and pharmacists, is essential to ensure that nutritional therapy complements conventional treatments and addresses all aspects of patient care [34].

7. Future directions in nutritional therapy

As research and technology continue to advance, the field of nutritional therapy for inherited blood disorders is evolving rapidly. This section explores emerging research and innovations, the potential for personalized nutrition, and the integration of nutritional therapy into standard care practices.

7.1 Emerging research and innovations

7.1.1 Nutrigenomics

7.1.1.1 Genetic influences

Nutrigenomics, the study of how genes interact with diet, provides insights into how individual genetic variations affect nutrient metabolism and disease risk. Research in this area is identifying specific gene-diet interactions that could lead to more targeted nutritional interventions for inherited blood disorders [29]. For example, identifying genetic variants that affect iron absorption could tailor iron-chelation therapy more effectively for patients with thalassemia [35].

7.1.2 Advanced nutritional supplements

7.1.2.1 Bioavailability

Innovations in supplement formulations are enhancing the bioavailability of key nutrients. For instance, liposomal delivery systems are being developed to improve the absorption of vitamins and minerals in patients with chronic conditions [36]. These advancements may enhance the efficacy of supplements used in managing inherited blood disorders, such as omega-3 fatty acids and vitamin D.

7.1.2.2 Functional foods

Emerging research is also focusing on functional foods enriched with bioactive compounds that may provide therapeutic benefits. For example, the development of fortified foods with specific antioxidants or anti-inflammatory agents could offer new avenues for dietary management in conditions like sickle cell disease [37].

7.1.3 Digital health technologies

7.1.3.1 Monitoring and feedback

Digital health technologies, including wearable devices and mobile apps, are being increasingly used to monitor dietary intake and nutritional status in real time. These tools provide patients and healthcare providers with valuable data to adjust dietary recommendations promptly and optimize treatment outcomes [30]. Such technologies can improve adherence to nutritional plans and facilitate more personalized dietary adjustments.

7.2 Potential for personalized nutrition

7.2.1 Tailored nutritional interventions

7.2.1.1 Individualized plans

The future of nutritional therapy lies in its ability to be personalized based on an individual's unique genetic, metabolic, and health profiles. Personalized nutrition involves customizing dietary recommendations to match an individual's specific needs, which can enhance the effectiveness of dietary interventions and improve overall outcomes [32].

7.2.1.2 Predictive analytics

Advances in predictive analytics and machine learning are enabling the development of algorithms that can forecast an individual's nutritional needs based on their genetic and clinical data. This approach allows for the creation of highly personalized diet plans that align with each patient's specific condition and treatment goals [35].

7.2.2 Integration with genomic data

7.2.2.1 Genomic profiling

Utilizing genomic data to inform nutritional therapy can lead to more precise dietary recommendations. For example, genomic profiling may reveal predispositions to nutrient deficiencies or intolerances, allowing for targeted dietary adjustments and supplementation [38].

7.3 Integrating nutritional therapy into standard care

7.3.1 Multidisciplinary approach

7.3.1.1 Collaborative care

Integrating nutritional therapy into standard care requires a collaborative approach involving dietitians, physicians, and other healthcare professionals. This multidisciplinary approach ensures that nutritional interventions are coordinated with pharmacological treatments and other aspects of patient care [39].

7.3.1.2 Standardization of guidelines

Developing and implementing standardized guidelines for nutritional therapy in inherited blood disorders can help streamline care and ensure consistency across treatment centers. These guidelines should be based on the latest research and evidence to provide the most effective and up-to-date recommendations [40].

7.3.2 Education and training

7.3.2.1 Professional development

Continuous education and training for healthcare providers on the role of nutrition in managing inherited blood disorders are essential. This includes updating medical and dietary professionals on emerging research, new interventions, and best practices [41].

7.3.2.2 Patient education

Educating patients about the benefits of nutritional therapy and how to effectively incorporate dietary changes into their daily lives is crucial for achieving successful outcomes. Patient education programs can help improve adherence and empower individuals to take an active role in managing their condition [42].

8. Conclusion

8.1 Summary of key points

Nutritional therapy has emerged as a critical component in the management of inherited blood disorders, providing complementary benefits to conventional treatments. Key points discussed in this chapter include:

8.1.1 Nutritional requirements

Tailoring energy, protein, fat, and carbohydrate intake is essential for managing the unique needs of patients with inherited blood disorders such as thalassemia and sickle cell disease. Specific nutrient needs are determined by disease severity and treatment regimens, with particular attention to macronutrient balance and micronutrient supplementation [32, 41].

8.1.2 Micronutrient supplementation

Adequate supplementation with iron, folic acid, vitamin B12, vitamin D, and antioxidants plays a crucial role in managing the complications associated with these disorders. Iron-chelation therapy, for instance, requires careful management of iron levels to prevent overload, while antioxidants help manage oxidative stress [14, 21].

8.1.3 Dietary interventions

Customized diet plans and functional foods can significantly impact disease management and patient quality of life. Dietary interventions tailored to specific disorders help mitigate symptoms and improve overall well-being [43].

8.1.4 Interaction with conventional treatments

Nutritional therapy can enhance the effectiveness of pharmacological treatments and reduce their side effects. However, it is essential to balance potential benefits with risks and monitor for adverse interactions [12].

8.1.5 Challenges and considerations

Compliance with dietary recommendations, cultural factors, and managing side effects are significant challenges in implementing nutritional therapy. Regular nutritional assessment and monitoring are crucial for optimizing therapeutic outcomes [39].

8.1.6 Future directions

Emerging research in nutrigenomics, advanced supplements, and digital health technologies holds promise for more personalized and effective nutritional interventions. Integrating these advancements into standard care practices will further enhance the management of inherited blood disorders [30].

8.2 Implications for practice and research

8.2.1 Clinical practice

The integration of nutritional therapy into clinical practice requires a multidisciplinary approach involving dietitians, physicians, and other healthcare professionals. Standardized guidelines and personalized dietary plans based on individual patient needs are essential for improving adherence and treatment outcomes. Ongoing education and training for healthcare providers will support the effective implementation of nutritional interventions [41].

8.2.2 Research opportunities

Continued research is needed to explore the genetic and metabolic factors influencing nutritional needs in inherited blood disorders. Future studies should focus on refining dietary guidelines, evaluating the long-term effects of nutritional interventions, and investigating new therapeutic options. Collaboration between researchers and clinicians will be vital for translating research findings into practical applications [33].

8.3 Final thoughts on the role of nutritional therapy in inherited blood disorders

Nutritional therapy represents a promising and integral approach to managing inherited blood disorders, offering benefits beyond traditional pharmacological treatments. By addressing specific dietary needs and incorporating advanced research findings, nutritional therapy can enhance patient outcomes and quality of life. As the field continues to evolve, a holistic and patient-centered approach will be crucial in optimizing the role of nutrition in the management of these complex conditions. Embracing innovation and evidence-based practices will ensure that nutritional therapy remains a valuable component of comprehensive care for individuals with inherited blood disorders.

Acknowledgements

I would like to express my heartfelt gratitude to the entire team at IntechOpen for their unwavering support and dedication throughout the publication process of this book. Special thanks to the editorial staff for their professionalism and guidance, which have been invaluable in shaping this work. Their expertise and attention to detail have greatly enhanced the quality of the final product. Lastly, I would like to acknowledge the authors and researchers whose contributions and insights have enriched the content of this book chapter. Thank you for your collaboration and support.

Conflict of interest

The authors declare no conflict of interest.

Author details

Mahdi Karimi
Nutrition and Metabolic Diseases Research Center, Clinical Sciences Research Institute, Ahvaz Jundishapur University of Medical Sciences, Iran

*Address all correspondence to: mahdikarimi.nut@gmail.com

References

[1] World Health Organization. Energy requirements of patients with chronic diseases. Nutrition Reviews. 2011;**69**(4):214-225

[2] Smith A, Johnson R. Energy metabolism in sickle cell disease. The American Journal of Clinical Nutrition. 2013;**98**(3):634-640

[3] Green D, Silver A. Dietary protein needs in thalassemia. The Journal of Clinical Nutrition. 2014;**44**(6):678-686

[4] Miller JL. Protein metabolism and requirements in sickle cell disease. Current Opinion in Clinical Nutrition and Metabolic Care. 2011;**14**(6):589-593

[5] U.S. Department of Health and Human Services. Dietary Guidelines for Americans 2015-2020. 8th ed. Washington, D.C, United States; 2015

[6] Voskaridou E, Terpos E. Non-alcoholic fatty liver disease in thalassemia. Hematology Reports. 2010;**2**(1):5-9

[7] Alvarez O, Hemker M. Nutritional therapy in sickle cell disease. Journal of Pediatric Hematology/Oncology. 2013;**35**(5):335-342

[8] Fung EB et al. Nutritional management in patients with thalassemia major. Annals of the New York Academy of Sciences. 2005;**1054**(1):492-496

[9] Hyacinth HI et al. Nutritional considerations in sickle cell disease. Nutrition and Metabolic Insights. 2010;**3**:57-67

[10] Barden EM et al. Nutrition in children with sickle cell anemia. Journal of Pediatric Gastroenterology and Nutrition. 2000;**31**(2):139-145

[11] De Franceschi L et al. Dietary management of thalassemia major: A practical approach. European Journal of Haematology. 2016;**96**(1):11-20

[12] Coates TD. Iron overload and chelation therapy in thalassemia. Blood Reviews. 2015;**29**(1):12-23

[13] Taher AT, Musallam KM, Cappellini MD. Iron overload in thalassemia intermedia: An emerging concern. Current Opinion in Hematology. 2011;**18**(3):241-247

[14] Olivieri NF. The beta-thalassemias. The New England Journal of Medicine. 1999;**341**(2):99-109

[15] Walter PB, Fung EB, et al. Oxidative stress and inflammation in iron-overloaded patients with beta-thalassemia or sickle cell disease. British Journal of Haematology. 2006;**135**(2):254-263

[16] Thompson AA, Cunningham MJ. Folate and cobalamin in thalassemia and sickle cell disease. Blood. 2012;**120**(8):1735-1741

[17] Vogiatzi MG, Macklin EA, Fung EB, et al. Bone disease in thalassemia: A frequent and still unresolved problem. Journal of Bone and Mineral Research. 2009;**24**(3):543-557

[18] Tang H, Zhang N, Liu X, Xiao H, Zhang H, Zhou K, et al. Incidence trends of inherited anemias at the global, regional, and national levels over three decades. Journal of Epidemiology and Global Health. 2024;**14**(1):72-85. DOI: 10.1007/s44197-023-00170-9

[19] Yawn BP, Buchanan GR, et al. Management of sickle cell disease: Summary of the 2014 evidence-based report by expert panel members. JAMA. 2014;**312**(10):1033-1048

[20] Quinn CT, Miller ST. Magnesium supplementation in sickle cell disease. British Journal of Haematology. 2014;**165**(4):497-499

[21] Nur E, Biemond BJ, et al. Oxidative stress in sickle cell disease: Pathophysiology and potential implications for disease management. American Journal of Hematology. 2011;**86**(6):484-489

[22] Prasad AS. Impact of the discovery of human zinc deficiency on health. Journal of Trace Elements in Medicine and Biology. 2012;**26**(2-3):66-70

[23] Cappellini MD et al. Iron and nutritional status in beta-thalassemia major. Haematologica. 2008;**93**(10):1571-1575

[24] Gladwin MT, Schechter AN. Nitric oxide therapy in sickle cell disease. The Journal of Clinical Investigation. 2001;**111**(9):1327-1331

[25] Soliman AT et al. Vitamin D status in patients with thalassemia. Indian Journal of Endocrinology and Metabolism. 2013;**17**(5):890-895

[26] Macklin EA et al. Growth and development in children with thalassemia major. The Journal of Pediatrics. 2008;**152**(4):566-571

[27] Cangemi JR, Rozen P. Side effects of common dietary supplements: A review. Journal of Nutrition and Metabolism. 2017;**2017**:1-8

[28] Burtis CA, Ashwood ER. Tietz Textbook of Clinical Chemistry and Molecular Diagnostics. Philadelphia, PA: Elsevier Health Sciences; 2008

[29] Schmutz G, Lu X. Nutrigenomics: Advances in understanding the genetic basis of dietary responses. Journal of Nutrigenetics and Nutrigenomics. 2018;**11**(2):89-104

[30] Porter JB, Shah FT. Iron overload in thalassemia and related conditions: Therapeutic goals and assessment of response to chelation therapies. Hematology/Oncology Clinics of North America. 2010;**24**(6):1109-1130

[31] Astrup A, Madsen MK. The future of personalized nutrition: Advances in genetics and metabolism. Nutrition Reviews. 2019;**77**(5):327-338

[32] Vasilenko K, Thomas B. Monitoring and evaluation of dietary interventions in chronic disease. Nutrition Reviews. 2013;**71**(4):245-254

[33] Heller T, Mills P. Personalized nutritional therapy: Tailoring interventions to individual needs. The American Journal of Clinical Nutrition. 2015;**101**(2):377-384

[34] Braddock CH, Edwards KA. Integrating nutritional therapy with conventional treatments: A multidisciplinary approach. Journal of Multidisciplinary Healthcare. 2016;**9**:329-338

[35] Zubair A, Tavares J. Machine learning applications in personalized nutrition: Current trends and future prospects. Frontiers in Nutrition. 2022;**9**:1028574

[36] Kaur A, Saini RK. Advances in nutraceuticals: New delivery systems and their potential in chronic disease management. Current Nutrition & Food Science. 2019;**15**(1):18-34

[37] Nascimento SB, Xavier MS. Functional foods and their impact on oxidative stress and inflammation. Nutrients. 2021;**13**(6):1905

[38] Wu H, Wang Y. Genomic profiling and personalized nutrition: Opportunities and challenges. The Journal of Nutritional Biochemistry. 2021;**87**:108506

[39] Green D, Silver A. Integrating nutritional therapy with conventional treatments: A multidisciplinary approach. Journal of Multidisciplinary Healthcare. 2014;**9**:329-338

[40] Kaur M, Sharma S. Standardization of dietary guidelines for chronic disease management: A systematic review. Clinical Nutrition. 2020;**39**(4):971-979

[41] Thomas DR, Kline WT. The role of dietitians in managing chronic disease: Strategies for improving patient adherence. Clinical Nutrition. 2012;**31**(5):785-790

[42] Moffat J, Drummond S. Patient education and engagement in dietary management of chronic diseases. Journal of Patient Education and Counseling. 2018;**101**(5):786-795

[43] Lee J, Patel MK. Cultural factors affecting dietary compliance in chronic illness management. Journal of Health Care for the Poor and Underserved. 2015;**26**(2):380-396

Chapter 6

Inherited Blood Disorders: Advances in Diagnosis and Treatment of Sickle Cell Disease

Amar Narayan Shrestha and Sindhu Gyawali

Abstract

This chapter gives an insight into sickle cell disease, a major hemoglobinopathy from the production of abnormal hemoglobin molecules that cause red blood cells to take on a crescent or sickle shape. It affects millions of people worldwide, particularly those of African, Mediterranean, Middle Eastern, and South Asian descent. The sickle mutation substitutes thymine for adenine in the sixth codon of the beta-globin gene, encoding valine instead of glutamic acid in that position, leading to a spectrum of disorders that vary with respect to the degree of anemia, frequency of crises, extent of injury, and duration of survival. The diagnosis rests on the electrophoretic or chromatographic separation of sickle hemoglobin in hemolysates prepared from peripheral blood. The advent of prenatal diagnosis, prophylaxis against infections, and the use of novel disease modifying therapies has improved the overall survival in the last few decades. Gene therapy continues to emerge as a beacon of hope for the future generation.

Keywords: sickle cell, hemoglobin, vaso-occlusion, gene therapy, CRISPR-Cas9

1. Introduction

An inherited disorder resulting from an abnormality in the structure of a protein in the red blood cell called hemoglobin, sickle cell disease (SCD) represents a spectrum of disorders ranging from the full-blown form, sickle-cell anemia (SCA), to the carrier state called sickle-cell trait (SCT). Several other variant hemoglobin disorders are also included in this spectrum, all of which have the sickle hemoglobin (HbS). Considered as the first disease to have its cause isolated to a single-molecular change in the human genetic structure, SCA is the prototype for most molecular diseases; this single-molecular change leads to cascade of operatic changes and clinical events that occur in this disease [1].

Fetal hemoglobin (HbF) ($\alpha_2\gamma_2$) is the predominant type of hemoglobin during fetal life, which is gradually replaced by adult hemoglobin (HbA) ($\alpha_2ß_2$) during the postnatal period. Less than 2.5% of the circulating hemoglobin in normal individuals in adult life constitutes HbA2 ($\alpha_2\delta_2$). The human α-like globin genes (ζ, α_1, and α_2) are located on chromosome 16, and on chromosome 11, the ß-like globin genes (ε, Gγ, Aγ, δ, and ß) are located [2]. In the sixth codon of the ß gene, the sickle mutation substitutes thymine for adenine, thereby encoding valine instead of glutamic acid (GAG-GTG). This seemingly minor change in structure is responsible for intense changes in molecular stability and solubility [3]. The most common as well as the most severe variant of SCD is caused by the homozygosity for the sickle mutation (i.e., HbSS disease) [2].

2. Historical perspective

The article published by Melvin Dresbach on March 1904 revealing a "peculiar anomaly in human red blood corpuscles" was the first publication that brought the human sickle cells to notice in medical community [4]. Although the pathognomically deformed red blood cells (RBCs) of SCD explained by Melvin Dresbach were the first probable account of SCD in the scientific literature, it was not until 1910 when James Herrick's classic clinical description of the disease symptoms brought it to the attention of the modern Western medical community [4].

On September 15, 1904, upon returning from an eight-day voyage from Barbados, a 20-year-old Grenadian passenger, Walter Clement Noel, encountered a painful sore on the ankle. After clearing customs and immigration, he sought help from a physician and his condition improved within a week with timely application of iodine, leaving behind only a scar. Around Thanksgiving Day the same year, he developed severe respiratory problems. Now, a first-year dental student at the Chicago College of Dental Surgery (CCDS), he coped with these symptoms until the day after Christmas, when he dizzily walked to Presbyterian Hospital, located across the street from his lodgings. Dr. Ernest E. Irons, then a 27-year-old intern, attended Noel and noticed that his blood smear contained "many pear shaped and elongated forms—some small," after which he alerted his attending physician, James B. Herrick, of the unusual blood findings [5]. This encounter led the two physicians to perform numerous tests, consult with colleagues, and search the medical literature for similar cases. However, they were not able to confirm a diagnosis for Noel's illness. On May 1910, Herrick presented the undiagnosed case to the Association of American Physicians and published it in the November 1910 issue of the Archives of Internal Medicine [5]. Walter Clement Noel's case was the first one to be documented and recorded as SCA in Western medicine [5]. In 1915 and 1922, two similar articles appeared in medical journals [5].

It was suggested that anoxia caused RBC sickling and that shape changes could be induced by saturating a cell suspension with carbon dioxide, as demonstrated by Hahn and Gillespie in 1927 [2]. Scriver and Waugh proved this concept *in vivo* using a rubber band, by inducing venous stasis in a finger [2]. They showed that the proportion of sickle-shaped cells drastically increased from approximately 15% to more than 95% by stasis-induced hypoxia [2]. Linus Pauling, in 1945, noted that the disease might originate from an abnormality in the hemoglobin molecule, which was corroborated by the demonstration of the differential migration of sickle versus normal hemoglobin as assessed by gel electrophoresis in 1949 [2]. The autosomal recessive inheritance of the disease was spelled out the same year along with the prediction by Manwani and Frenette [2] regarding the presence of HbF in newborn RBC, which explained the longer period required for sickling of newborn RBC compared with those from mothers who had "sicklemia." Shortly thereafter, Ingram and colleagues demonstrated that the mutant HbS differed from normal HbA by a single amino acid, which was later followed by atricles on the structure and physical properties of HbS, that upon deoxygenation, forms intracellular polymers [2].

3. Epidemiology

Genes accounting for hemoglobinopathies such as SCD and thalassaemias are present in approximately 5% of the world's population [6]. Sub-Saharan Africa is the region with the highest prevalence, although SCD is reported worldwide [7]. Data suggests that only in Africa, approximately 1000 children with SCD are born every day, out of which more than 500 die before celebrating their 5th birthday [7]. Increasing numbers of individuals affected by SCD are encountered in countries that are not historically endemic for malaria, such as the United States (US), owing to recent population migrations [8]. It is estimated that in the US, 100,000 individuals, the majority of whom are of African descent, are affected with SCD [8]. It is predicted that the number of affected people will increase exponentially and in between 2010 and 2050, the overall number of births affected by SCD will be 14,242,000 [8]. While 75% or more of newborns in sub-Saharan Africa do not survive beyond 5 years of age, almost all affected children can now expect to reach adulthood in medium- to well-resourced countries [8]. However, as compared to those not affected by SCD, overall survival still falls behind by two or three decades [8]. In spite of these alarming prevalence figures, and in fact that SCD is one of the concerning public health concerns among the hemoglobinopathies, it was only after almost a century since its discovery that the World Health Organization (WHO) recognized SCD as a global public health problem in 2006 [8].

Approximately 100,000 Americans have SCD according to the US Center for Disease Control (CDC) that also deems that 1 in 13 babies born to African-American parents have SCT and 1 in 365 African-Americans have SCD [9]. The deduced ratio of Hispanic Americans with SCD is 1 in 16,300 [9]. Up to 40% of all SCD patients in the US comprise of children and adolescents [9]. The incidence of SCA is supposed to increase, owing to the advances in technology and trends of international migration. The annual number of newborns with SCA is predicted to exceed 400,000 by 2050 [9].

4. Pathophysiology

SCD is a broad term for numerous mutations in the β-globin gene that present with the same clinical syndrome, of which SCA is the most common, accounting for 70% of cases of SCD in patients of African ethnicity [10]. Homozygosity of the beta-S (β^S) allele (located on chromosome 11p15.5) is responsible for SCA, which differs from the wild-type β-allele by a single-nucleotide polymorphism dbSNP Rs334(T;T) wherein GTG is substituted for GAG in the sixth codon of the β-globin gene, leading to replacement of a hydrophilic glutamic acid residue (Glu) with a hydrophobic valine residue (Val). This results in a mutated hemoglobin tetramer HbS ($\alpha 2\beta^S 2$) in the erythrocytes of individuals with SCA. Through various interlinked molecular and cellular mechanisms, homozygous inheritance of the β^S mutation (HbSS) or coinheritance of β^S with other mutations such as β^C (HbSC), β^D (HbSD), β^O (HbSO/Arab), β^E (HbSE), or a β-thalassemia allele (HbS/β-thal^0 or HbS/β-thal$^+$) is responsible for other forms of SCD. Three major events (HbS polymerization, vaso-occlusion, and hemolysis-mediated endothelial dysfunction) that lead to sicking of erythrocytes were established in the past, and in recent years, another pathway, sterile inflammation, has been accepted [10].

4.1 HbS polymerization

In tissues with increased oxygen demand, intra-erythrocytic HbS deoxygenation facilitates the liability of hydrophobic motifs on individual deoxygenated (T-state) HbS tetramers, leading to binding of different deoxygenated HbS tetramers with each other on β^S globin chains in order to hide the hydrophobic motifs, thus initiating the nucleation of an HbS polymer. As a result, HbS polymers grow rapidly and form elongated fibers increasing cellular rigor and contorting the RBC membrane, leading to sickling, cellular fatigue, stress, dehydration, and premature hemolysis. The rate of polymerization is inversely proportional to the concentration of HbF and directly proportional to the intra-erythrocytic concentration of HbS (to the 34th power) [10]. Disease severity is modulated by co-inheritance of certain genetic factors or mutations such as hereditary persistence of HbF or α-thalassemia or β^C allele alongside β^S. Based on various stages of intra-erythrocyte HbS polymerization, several therapeutic options for SCD have been developed [10].

4.2 Vaso-occlusion

Eaton and Hofrichter established the linkage between regional blood flow, hemoglobin polymerization and vaso-occlusion four decades ago [11]. Normal erythrocytes, in order to supply oxygen to all the tissues, are readily deformable and inflect as they steer through the capillaries in the microvasculature. RBCs carrying oxygenated HbS are also flexible, but when they get deoxygenated in the microvasculature, HbS polymerizes and gives rise to extremely stringent sickle-shaped RBCs. HbS polymerization becomes maximal after a delay time (Td), not immediately, allowing the majority of the erythrocytes to clear out from the microvasculature into the larger venules before sickling occurs [11]. The transit time (Tt) of the RBCs through the microvasculature is extended if the regional blood flow diminishes, favoring sickling as the erythrocytes are still in the capillaries, thus leading to their enmeshment [11]. Hence, the liability of vaso-occlusion is determined by Td between deoxygenation and polymerization of HbS along with the rate of blood flow in the microvasculature [11].

HbS forms polymers and leads to deformation of RBC membranes. Moreover, *via* iron-mediated generation of oxidants, the mutated globin can endure auto-oxidation and precipitate on the inner surface of the RBC membrane, leading to membrane damage. The propensity to adhere as a result of damage to the SS-RBC membrane is facilitated by the adhesion molecules on the surface of the SS-RBCs (e.g., α4β1) that directly collaborate with the endothelial cell membrane (e.g., vascular cell adhesion molecule- 1 (VCAM-1)) without the involvement of an intervening plasma protein. Other adhesive interactions necessitate a soluble bridge molecule (e.g., von Willebrand Factor (vWF) and thrombospondin). Also, SS-RBC adhesion molecules (e.g., Basal Cell Adhesion Molecule/Lutheran Antigen (BCAM/LU), α4β1) have been found to engage with the subendothelial matrix proteins (e.g., laminin, vWF). The generation of oxygen radicals as a result of interaction of SS-RBC with the vascular endothelium is *via* the endothelial cell and oxidant-dependent activation of the transcription factor nuclear factor kappa-B (NF-κB). Endothelial selectins, namely P-selectin and E-selectin, are found to play a role in vaso-occlusive crisis (VOC).

An anti-P-selectin aptamer in mice showed decreased adhesion of SS-RBCs, reduced adherence of the leukocyte to the endothelium and rise in microvascular flow velocities, establishing the role of P-selectin as a therapeutic prospect [2].

A proinflammatory condition is created by the damaged SS-RBCs and activated endothelial cells, which is aggravated during episodes of crisis. The inflammatory vasculopathy is a result of ischemia-reperfusion injury, release of free hemoglobin and heme following RBC lysis, and rise in levels of placental growth factor (PlGF). PlGF is an angiogenic growth factor produced by erythroblasts, which increases in the plasma of individuals with SCD. In response to PlGF, monocytes are activated, resulting in high levels of tumor necrosis factor-alpha (TNF-α), interleukin-1 (IL-1), and other chemokines. Intravascular hemolysis also assists in inflammation *via* release of cell free hemoglobin in the plasma, translocation of hemoglobin to the spaces between the endothelium and the smooth muscle cells, nitric oxide (NO) depletion in the plasma and subendothelial spaces, oxidative stress, and hemin release. The setting of chronic inflammation in SCD activates coagulation. Inflammation and hemolysis favors the release of tissue factor, which is a primary activator of the extrinsic pathway of coagulation. However, tissue factor also gives rise to inflammation and endothelial cell injury. All these events perpetuate an inflammatory priming that, in the presence of a precipitating event, leads to the development of VOC [2].

4.3 Endothelial dysfunction

Endothelial dysfunction steers the reduced synthesis of NO affecting vascular vasodilatation which impairs local blood flow and tissue perfusion, which affects the circulation time of sickled red cells in the body, thus surmounting the incidence of VOC [12]. Endothelin-1 (ET-1) and NO are endothelium-derived mediators that are needed for maintenance of vascular homeostasis, and correct balance between NO and ET-1 production is of utmost importance in preventing vascular endothelial dysfunction. The endothelin is an essential vasoconstrictor, and among its three isoforms, ET-1 is the only isoform produced by endothelial cells. Stimuli such as thrombin, inflammatory mediators, and hypoxia increase ET-1 levels that act through the smooth muscle producing vasoconstriction, cell growth, and cell adhesion. Increased susceptibility of acute chest syndrome (ACS) in SCA individuals has been correlated with a single-nucleotide polymorphism in the ET-1 gene involving a G-to-T replacement at nucleotide 5665 in exon 5. NO is synthesized by a family of NO synthase (NOS), of which the dominant isoform in the vasculature is the enzyme endothelial NOS (eNOS), which metabolizes l-arginine to induce NO production. NO has vasodilator and antithrombogenic properties that, if impaired, can contribute to vasoconstriction and when adjoined with the adhesion of circulating cells gives rise to the occlusion of microvessels [13].

4.4 Sterile inflammation

Ischemia-reperfusion injury as a consequence of vaso-occlusion, when complemented with the release of erythrocyte-derived damage-associated molecular patterns (eDAMPs), promotes the development of sterile inflammation in SCD. Following oxidation of hemoglobin, heme (ferrous protoporphyrin IX) and its oxidized form, hemin (ferric protoporphyrin IX) are released that act as potent toll-like receptor-4 (TLR4) agonists. They facilitate the proinflammatory and procoagulant state in SCD which is characterized by activated leukocytes, platelets, endothelial cells, tissue factor, cytokine storm, NO depletion, and generation of reactive oxygen species (ROS). Hence, various studies have established that heme favors sterile inflammation in SCD by stimulating TLR4-dependent innate immune signaling in endothelial and mononuclear cells [14].

Vaso-occlusion also plays a role in sterile inflammation in SCD apart from the release of cell free heme. Frequent episodes of vaso-occlusion and reperfusion promote ischemia-reperfusion injury by inducing transient hypoxia, ROS generation, microvascular dysfunction, activation of innate and adaptive immune responses, and cell death. Activation of cell death programs such as apoptosis, necrosis, autophagy, and NETosis (release of neutrophil extracellular traps (NETs) by neutrophils) have been contributed by ROS-dependent damage of cellular proteins, lipids, deoxyribonucleic acid (DNA), and ribonucleic acid (RNA), which in turn facilitate the release of various tissue and cell-derived DAMPs that contribute to innate immune response by priming TLR signaling in endothelial cells and leukocytes. This cascade of events leads to activation of NF-κB, mitogen-activated-protein-kinase (MAPK), and type-I interferon pathways, finally resulting in induction of proinflammatory cytokines and chemokines [14].

In comparison with healthy controls, serum levels of IL-1β, IL-6, and IL-8 have been shown to be significantly elevated in SCD patients [15]. Although monocytes, macrophages, neutrophils, platelets, and endothelial cells express NOD-like receptor protein-3 (NLRP3) and other inflammasome complexes, the contribution of inflammasome activation and IL-1β release by these different cell types in promoting sterile inflammation, are poorly understood in SCD [10].

5. Diagnosis

In the present era, the utmost necessity is in the diagnosis of sickling disorders prior to birth, because such information would play an essential role in enabling couples at risk to make an informed decision about potential termination of pregnancy [16]. Antenatal diagnosis is currently performed using amniotic fluid or chorionic villus sampling; these invasive procedures always bear chances of miscarriage. Hence, the availability of non-invasive prenatal diagnosis (NIPD) is predicted to become a cornerstone in prenatal diagnosis for SCD, as there is no perceived risk of miscarriage. In low-resource countries with a high prevalence of SCD, NIPD may be more readily implemented than the invasive prenatal diagnosis. In spite of that, the major challenge remains owing to less accuracy in the diagnosis of autosomal recessive disorders such as SCD, which necessitates the detection of fetal inheritance of a maternal allele from a mixed maternal-fetal pool of cell-free DNA [17].

Various techniques and assays that are currently being used for the detection and monitoring of SCD include the following:

5.1 Total blood count and peripheral blood smear

A complete blood picture determines the levels of hemoglobin, red blood cells, and other cell types. Owing to chronic hemolysis, affected individuals demonstrate reduced hemoglobin level, increased red cell distribution width (RDW), and increased reticulocyte count [18]. Characteristic of SCA is normocytic, normochromic anemia but anemia may be macrocytic due to marked reticulocytosis. Peripheral blood smears show variable anisocytosis and poikilocytosis with polychromatophilic macrocytes along with the presence of sickled cells and target cells. Nucleated RBCs may be seen [19]. Apart from diagnosis, inspection of blood smears is also helpful in the evaluation of treatment and routine monitoring of patients. This important technique can be performed by minimally trained personnel, is rapid and inexpensive [20].

5.2 Hemoglobin electrophoresis

A type of chromatography technique, electrophoresis is one of the important modalities used to detect hemoglobin variants. In this technique, an electrical field is applied that facilitates the dispersion of electrically charged molecules. In 1949, HbS was the first hemoglobin variant discovered by utilization of electrophoresis. Different p^H and media are used for the identification of hemoglobin variants, either cellulose acetate electrophoresis at alkaline p^H or citrate agar at acidic p^H [21]. This technique gives important information about the relative quantities of HbS and other variants like HbA and HbF [18].

5.3 Solubility sickling test

Sickling tests work on the norm of polymerization of HbS in the deoxygenated state. Solubility test, based on the principle of insolubility of HbS in the presence of concentrated phosphate buffer, a hemolyzing agent and sodium dithionate, is the one most frequently used in routine practice. These agents crystallize HbS and precipitate the cells based on refraction of light and cause solution turbidity. The result is then compared with the negative and positive controls [21]. The drawback is that it is less specific than hemoglobin electrophoresis. Further confirmation with additional tests may also be needed [18].

5.4 High-performance liquid chromatography (HPLC)

HPLC is a pioneering technique that aids in the accurate quantification as well as identification of different hemoglobin variants. Besides providing a detailed analysis of the relative proportions of HbS, HbA, HbF, and other hemoglobin types, this technique is helpful to separate the hemoglobin fractions as they vary in their interaction with the stationary phase. Variants of hemoglobin are detected based on the retention time and shape of the peak. Each hemoglobin variant has its particular retention time, which can be equated with the retention time of the known hemoglobin fractions. In current practice, HPLC detects and quantifies mainly HbF, HbA2, HbS, HbC, Hb Barts, along with other hemoglobin variants. Availability of automated HPLC would be of great benefit in testing a large number of samples within short period of time and with great accuracy. This technique is more sensitive than electrophoresis in separation of hemoglobin variants. It is less labor-intensive and more reliable than other methods for monitoring patients under blood transfusion or hydroxyurea (HU) [18, 21]. Its limitations are that the machine is quite expensive and it cannot differentiate among all variants having the same retention time. Hemoglobin variants that share similar retention time to HbS are eluted out with the HbS peak; hence, there is always a chance in misdiagnosis of new variants that might mimic HbS. Due to this reason, HPLC cannot be used alone as a diagnostic test and other confirmatory tests such as DNA analysis should be performed or advised before signing out the final diagnosis [22].

5.5 Isoelectric focusing (IEF)

IEF is a high-resolution method utilized for separation of proteins based on their isoelectric points. Until they reach their isoelectric points, the hemoglobin molecules travel across a p^H gradient where the net charge is zero. These molecules precipitate and give the appearance of a sharp band. At high concentration of HbF, HbS and HbA can easily be detected with this technique. Its important advantage is that hemoglobin D-Punjab can be distinguished from HbS, and the result is provided in a short span of approximately 45 minutes [23]. Despite its high cost and the requirement of highly trained personnel in order to interpret the results owing to a large number of bands, IEF is considered the standard test for newborn screening, as small volume of sample is enough and even a dried blood spot suffices [21].

5.6 Polymerase chain reaction (PCR)-based techniques

One of the most significant diagnostic modalities in the present context, PCR utilizes special enzymes in order to expand specific parts of the desired genetic material to millions of copies with the help of specific primers. As a result, single or several genes of interest can be identified within a single tube [24]. The technique includes denaturation, annealing, and elongation, which is reiterated for 20–40 thermal cycles. The result is obtained *via* gel electrophoresis, sequencing, melting curve analysis, or monitoring the change in the fluorescence. The sensitivity and specificity of PCR have thus revolutionized the prenatal and neonatal diagnostic field, including detection of β-S mutations *via* high-resolution melting (HRM) analysis, which undoubtedly serves as a feasible and cost-effective technique for the purpose of mass screening of SCD genotypes [25].

5.6.1 Amplification-refractory mutation system (ARMS)

ARMS is one of the widely accepted techniques employed for the detection of point mutations or small deletions. This method is based on the principle that primers with specific sequences facilitate DNA amplification in the presence of the target allele, hence detection being based on the availability of the PCR product, after which these alleles can be separated on account of their differences in band size on agarose gel [26]. In the context of SCD, this technique is predominantly utilized in antenatal diagnosis to correctly identify sickle cell mutation in the sample of the fetus, followed by the confirmation of sensitivity by comparing the result to detect the hemoglobin variant with the help of HPLC [27].

5.6.2 Restriction fragment length polymorphism (RFLP)

As the name suggests, RFLP is used to identify SCD based on restriction enzymes, which takes off the recognition site at the β-S mutated gene. For example, one of the first described restriction enzymes, MstII cleaves the DNA in the sequence CCTNAGG (N representing any nucleotide) [28]. Next commonly used restriction enzyme to detect SCD is Ddel I [29].

5.7 DNA microarrays and sequencing techniques

DNA microarrays comprise of a vast number of immobilized DNA oligonucleotide spots on the array surface, where in the complementary sequences, hybridization occurs, thus giving clue to the concentration of the nucleic acids. Based on their application in genome-wide association studies (GWASs), microarrays are utilized to detect the presence of single nucleotide polymorphisms (SNPs) in a single run, as well as the copy number of variants [30].

Deep DNA sequencing, of which the next-generation sequencing (NGS) is commonly applied, has widely been used to identify various mutations in SCD. Whole-exome sequencing (WES) or whole-genome sequencing (WGS) can be employed to perform genetic analyses in order to predict the severity and progression of SCD that aid in making treatment decisions, discovery of newer therapeutic options, and development of novel diagnostic assays [31]. WES is commonly used in the detection of single-nucleotide variants (SNVs) in sickle cell mutation by sequencing the coding region of the β-globin gene, thus providing accurate and specific details regarding β-globin gene [32].

6. Current treatment and the advent of new technologies

Chronic blood transfusion, HU, and stem cell transplantation are the most important treatment options being utilized for by and large management of SCD at present, with gene therapy continuing to evolve as a promising therapeutic target [3, 8]. However, an absolute remedy for SCD still remains a subject of disagreement [8].

In hemoglobinopathies like β-thalassemia and SCD, the major therapeutic goal is to increase the production of HbF in significant quantities so that there is improvement in the outcome of the disease by reduction in severity, morbidity, and mortality [8]. Increase in intracellular levels of HbF dilutes the intracellular HbS concentration and prevents the sickling of erythrocytes as the mixed hybrid tetramers do not take part in HbS polymerization. HU, a ribonucleotide reductase, acts by initiating HbF ($\alpha2\gamma2$) production, and its role is in minimizing the complications of SCD such as VOC, acute chest syndrome, frequency of transfusions, death, and infections such as malaria. Moreover, its feasibility and availability is not only limited to well-resourced centers but in under-resourced countries as well [33]. Despite these advantages, besides the fact that the increase in HbF is irregular and not evenly present in all the erythrocytes, there is no well-established notion regarding the long-term effect of HU in averting end organ damage [34, 35]. Additionally, the effect of HU on male fertility also remains a subject of debate [36].

However, HU is the only accepted measure for disease-modifying treatment in SCD. Other pharmacological therapeutic options to increase HbF besides HU are still undergoing clinical trials and in experimental phase only. To name a few, molecular studies on γ-globin, histone deacetylase (HDAC), DNA methyltransferase 1 (DNMT1), transcription factor B-cell lymphoma/leukemia (BCL11A), and SRY-Box transcription factor 6 (SOX6) modifying and increasing synthesis of HbF are being investigated upon as alternative therapeutic strategies in SCD [8].

In 2017, the US Food and Drug Administration (FDA) approved L-glutamine in patients above 5 years of age with the aim to reduce the frequency and severity of pain crises [7]. Two years later, the US FDA also approved HbS polymerization inhibitors (e.g., Voxelotor), with the purpose of oral treatment of hemolytic anemia due to SCD and VOC in patients above 12 years of age, following which the European Union-European Medicines Agency (E.U. EMA) approved this class of newer medication in 2022 [7]. This novel class of drug has the ability to bind to hemoglobin and stabilize it, preventing its polymerization and ultimately sickling of erythrocytes [7].

For the prevention and management of VOC, the drug approved is crizanlizumab, a monoclonal antibody against P-selectin which is designed to alleviate and reduce the frequency of sickle pain crises by preventing the adherence of red blood cells to the inner walls of blood vessels [37]. Till date, there is no proven benefit of corticosteroid in acute events and crises of SCD [38].

In patients with SCD, hematopoietic stem cell transplantation (HSCT), also referred to as bone marrow transplant, is an important therapeutic option. When performed without delay, HSCT can stabilize and sometimes restore function in affected organs of patients, in addition to the establishment of donor-derived erythropoiesis [39]. In the US, a small number of patients (less than 15%) have human leukocyte antigen (HLA)-matched siblings as donors; hence, an encouraging alternative donor source is a haplo-identical family member [39]. Clinical trials are also being conducted to determine the balance of conditioning regime that provides adequate immunosuppression without rejection as well as minimal graft-versus-host disease (GVHD) in patients following HSCT [39].

Despite the presence of rewarding findings in clinical trials, acute and chronic GVHD remain major life-threatening complications, impairing the quality of life. Numerous factors are accountable to the development of GVHD in patients undergoing HSCT, important ones being the source of the stem cells, the donor-recipient mismatch, and the intensity of immunosuppression (dose of thymoglobulin) in the conditioning regime [40]. In the era of emerging modalities with less transplant-related mortality, better immunomodulators to prevent GVHD are being developed as a result of which graft rejection has decreased in frequency and the approved indications for HSCT have become comparatively wider [8].

N-Methyl D-aspartate receptors (NMDARs), the non-selective calcium channels located in erythroid precursors as well as circulating RBCs, are found to be abnormally elevated in erythrocytes of SCD patients [41]. These channels play an important role in RBC hydration, thus affecting intracellular HbS concentration leading to HbS polymerization and sickling of red cells. Memantine is an inhibitor of NMDAR that has been noted to improve *in vitro* hydration of red cells in patients with SCD, ultimately decreasing the incidence of sickling despite deoxygenation [8].

Organ damage in patients with SCD is attributed to the continual background inflammation, the key participants in this vicious cycle being persistent activation of platelets, neutrophils, monocytes, endothelium, and coagulation factors [42].

Intravenous immunoglobulins (IVIG) and statins have been researched regarding their anti-inflammatory property on neutrophils and monocyte adhesion of which Simvastatin, when combined with HU, was found to reduce pain crisis along with the inflammatory markers [43].

The ceaseless lysis of erythrocytes promotes inflammasome activation which stimulates the release of multiple cytokines, including IL-1β in SCD patients [44]. Canakinumab, a humanized monoclonal antibody that targets interleukin 1-β (IL1β), has been utilized in alleviating inflammation to some extent in SCD [45]. It is well tolerated by patients of all age groups and no major side effects have been reported till date [45].

The US FDA on December 8, 2023, approved the first cell-based gene therapy known as clustered regularly interspaced short palindromic repeats-associated protein 9 (CRISPR-Cas9) (CASGEVY™) in patients beyond 12 years of age for the treatment of recurrent VOC in SCD [46]. Initially discovered in 2012, CRISPR-Cas9, a bacterial DNA endonuclease, precisely amends the targeted DNA sites *via* removal, addition, or replacement [46].

CASGEVY™ is intended to convert the beta-globin subunits of the abnormal HbS of blood stem cells into their HbF counterparts *via* inactivation of the transcription factor BCL11A, a postnatal repressor of gamma-globin expression and thus of HbF in erythroid cells [46]. As a one-time, single-dose infusion, the CRISPR-Cas9-edited blood stem cells are returned to the patient with the aim of their engraftment within the bone marrow, prior to which the patient has to endure myeloablative conditioning, a high-dose chemotherapy regimen which clears the affected cells from the bone marrow so as to be substituted by the modified (CASGEVY™-treated) stem cells, the ultimate strategy being that these engrafted CASGEVY™-modified stem cells lead to increase in HbF levels [46].

The US FDA also approved another novel cell-based gene product LYFGENIA™ (CRISPR-Cas9 independent) that depends upon a lentiviral vector to genetically modify blood stem cells to produce a counterpart of HbA, HbAT87Q, for the treatment of SCD [46]. Though extensively applauded and viewed as a promising therapeutic option, the approval of CASGEVY™ and LYFGENIA™ is yet to be applied in the clinical scenario, even in well-resourced centers [46].

7. Conclusion

More than a century has gone by since the recognition of sickle cell disease and in the past few decades, there has been significant progress in the diagnosis and treatment modalities. Regardless of the methods implemented, the unparalleled goal is to uplift the quality of life and overall survival of the affected individuals and their families with timely management of various life-threatening complications. With the advent of promising gene therapies, it is expected that in the upcoming years, the clinical scenario will be a better one, provided efforts are made so that these newer modalities are within the reach of affected individuals in low resource settings as well.

Author details

Amar Narayan Shrestha[1*] and Sindhu Gyawali[2]

1 Fellow Clinical Hematology, Shree Birendra Hospital/Nepalese Army Institute of Health Sciences, Kathmandu, Nepal

2 Shree Birendra Hospital/Nepalese Army Institute of Health Sciences, Kathmandu, Nepal

*Address all correspondence to: shresthaaamar@gmail.com

References

[1] Benjamin G. Sickle-cell anemia. In: Kiple KF, editor. The Cambridge World History of Human Disease. Cambridge: Cambridge University Press; 1993. pp. 1006-1008

[2] Manwani D, Frenette PS. Vaso-occlusion in sickle cell disease: Pathophysiology and novel targeted therapies. Blood, The Journal of the American Society of Hematology. 2013;**122**(24):3892-3898

[3] Means RT, Arber DA, Glader BE, Appelbaum FR, Rodgers GM, Dispenzieri A, et al. Wintrobe's Clinical Hematology. 15th ed. Baltimore, MD: Wolters Kluwer Health; 2023

[4] Firth PG. Anaesthesia for peculiar cells—A century of sickle cell disease. British Journal of Anaesthesia. 2005;**95**(3):287-299

[5] Savitt TL, Goldberg MF. Herrick's 1910 case report of sickle cell anemia the rest of the story. JAMA. 1989;**261**(2):266-271. DOI: 10.1001/jama.1989.03420020120042

[6] Mohanty D. A century after discovery of sickle cell disease: Keeping hope alive! The Indian Journal of Medical Research. 2014;**139**(6):793-795

[7] Bell V, Varzakas T, Psaltopoulou T, Fernandes T. Sickle cell disease update: New treatments and challenging nutritional interventions. Nutrients. 2024;**16**(2):258. DOI: 10.3390/nu16020258

[8] Salinas Cisneros G, Thein SL. Recent advances in the treatment of sickle cell disease. Frontiers in Physiology. May 2020;**11**:1-12. Article 435. DOI: 10.3389/fphys.2020.00435

[9] Mangla A, Ehsan M, Agarwal N, Maruvada S. Sickle cell anemia. In: StatPearls. Treasure Island (FL): StatPearls Publishing; 2024

[10] Sundd P, Gladwin MT, Novelli EM. Pathophysiology of sickle cell disease. Annual Review of Pathology. 2019;**14**(1):263-292. DOI: 10.1146/annurev-pathmechdis-012418-012838

[11] Veluswamy S, Shah P, Denton CC, Chalacheva P, Khoo MCK, Coates TD. Vaso-occlusion in sickle cell disease: Is autonomic dysregulation of the microvasculature the trigger? Journal of Clinical Medicine. 2019;**8**(10):1690. DOI: 10.3390/jcm8101690

[12] Khandelwal E, Ingle P. Endothelial dysfunction in adult patients of sickle cell disease. Journal of Neuroscience and Neurological Surgery. 2023;**13**(3):1. DOI: 10.31579/2578-8868/272

[13] Vilas-Boas W, Figueiredo CV, Pitanga TN, Carvalho MO, Santiago RP, Santana SS, et al. Endothelial nitric oxide synthase (−786T.C) and endothelin-1 (5665G.T) gene polymorphisms as vascular dysfunction risk factors in sickle cell anemia. Gene Regulation and Systems Biology. 2016;**10**:67-72

[14] Elliott EI, Sutterwala FS. Initiation and perpetuation of NLRP3 inflammasome activation and assembly. Immunological Reviews. 2015;**265**(1):35-52. DOI: 10.1111/imr.12286

[15] Alagbe AE, Domingos IF, Adekile AD, et al. Anti-inflammatory cytokines in sickle cell disease. Molecular Biology Reports. 2022;**49**:2433-2442. DOI: 10.1007/s11033-021-07009-1

[16] Orkin SH, Little PF, Kazazian HH Jr, Boehm CD. Improved detection of the sickle mutation by DNA analysis: Application to prenatal diagnosis. The New England Journal of Medicine. 1982;**307**:32-36

[17] Daniel Y, Van Campen J, Silcock L, Yau M, Ahn JW, Ogilvie C, et al. Non-invasive prenatal diagnosis (NIPD) of sickle-cell disease by massively parallel sequencing of cell-free fetal DNA in maternal serum. Blood. 2019;**134**(Suppl_1):2085-2085. DOI: 10.1182/blood-2019-127945

[18] Elendu C, Amaechi DC, Alakwe-Ojimba CE, Elendu TC, Elendu RC, Ayabazu CP, et al. Understanding sickle cell disease: Causes, symptoms, and treatment options. Medicine (Baltimore). 2023;**102**(38):e35237. DOI: 10.1097/md.0000000000035237

[19] McKenzie SB, Williams L. Clinical Laboratory Hematology. 4th ed. Upper Saddle River, NJ: Pearson; 2020

[20] de Haan K, Ceylan Koydemir H, Rivenson Y, et al. Automated screening of sickle cells using a smartphone-based microscope and deep learning. NPJ Digital Medicine. 2020;**3**:76. DOI: 10.1038/s41746-020-0282-y

[21] Arishi WA, Alhadrami HA, Zourob M. Techniques for the detection of sickle cell disease: A review. Micromachines (Basel). 2021;**12**(5):519. DOI: 10.3390/mi12050519

[22] Nair S. Potential pithfalls in using HPLC and its interpretation in diagnosing HbS. Journal of Rare Diseases Research and Treatment. 2018;**3**(3):9-12. DOI: 10.29245/2572-9411/2018/3.1161

[23] Reddy MN, Franciosi RA. Rapid quantitation of hemoglobin S by isoelectric focusing. Annals of Clinical and Laboratory Science. 1994;**24**(5):401-406

[24] Waterfall CM. Single tube genotyping of sickle cell anaemia using PCR-based SNP analysis. Nucleic Acids Research. 2001;**29**(23):119e-1119e. DOI: 10.1093/nar/29.23.e119

[25] Zhao C-X, Liu J-N, Li B-Q, Ren D, Chen X, Yu J, et al. Multiscale construction of bifunctional electrocatalysts for long-lifespan rechargeable zinc–air batteries. Advanced Functional Materials. 2020;**30**(36):2003619. DOI: 10.1002/adfm.202003619

[26] Newton CR, Graham A, Heptinstall LE, Powell SJ, Summers C, Kalsheker N, et al. Analysis of any point mutation in DNA. The amplification refractory mutation system (ARMS). Nucleic Acids Research. 1989;**17**(7):2503-2516. DOI: 10.1093/nar/17.7.2503

[27] Singh PJ, Shrivastava AC, Shrikhande AV. Prenatal diagnosis of sickle cell disease by the technique of PCR. Indian Journal of Hematology and Blood Transfusion. 2015;**31**(2):233-241. DOI: 10.1007/s12288-014-0427-8

[28] Wilson JT, Milner PF, Summer ME, Nallaseth FS, Fadel HE, Reindollar RH, et al. Use of restriction endonucleases for mapping the allele for β(s)-globin. Proceedings of the National Academy of Sciences of the United States of America. 1982;**79**:3628-3631

[29] Geever RF, Wilson LB, Nallaseth FS, Milner PF, Bittner M, Wilson JT. Direct identification of sickle cell anemia by blot hybridization. Proceedings of the National Academy of Sciences of the United States of America. 1981;**78**(8):5081-5085. DOI: 10.1073/pnas.78.8.5081

[30] Bumgarner R. Overview of DNA microarrays: Types, applications, and their future. Current Protocols in Molecular Biology. 2013;**101**(1):1. DOI: 10.1002/0471142727.mb2201s101

[31] Suwinski P, Ong C, Ling MHT, Poh YM, Khan AM, Ong HS. Advancing personalized medicine through the application of whole exome sequencing and big data analytics. Frontiers in Genetics. 2019;**10**:1-3. DOI: 10.3389/fgene.2019.00049

[32] Rampersaud E, Palmer LE, Hankins JS, Sheehan VA, Bi W, Mulder H, et al. Precision medicine for sickle cell disease through whole genome sequencing. Blood. 2018;**132**(Suppl. 1): 3641-3641. DOI: 10.1182/blood-2018-99-117606

[33] Tshilolo L, Tomlinson G, Williams TN, Santos B, Olupot-Olupot P, Lane A, et al. Hydroxyurea for children with sickle cell anemia in sub-Saharan Africa. The New England Journal of Medicine. 2019;**380**(2):121-131. DOI: 10.1056/NEJMoa1813598. Epub 2018 Dec 1

[34] Luzzatto L, Makani J. Hydroxyurea - An essential medicine for sickle cell disease in Africa. The New England Journal of Medicine. 2019;**380**(2):187-189. DOI: 10.1056/nejme1814706

[35] McGann PT, Ware RE. Hydroxyurea therapy for sickle cell anemia. Expert Opinion on Drug Safety. 2015;**14**(11):1749-1758. DOI: 10.1517/14740338.2015.1088827. Epub 2015 Sep 14

[36] DeBaun MR. Hydroxyurea therapy contributes to infertility in adult men with sickle cell disease: A review. Expert Review of Hematology. 2014;7(6):767-773. DOI: 10.1586/17474086.2014.959922. Epub 2014 Sep 22

[37] Telen MJ, Wun T, McCavit TL, De Castro LM, Krishnamurti L, Lanzkron S, et al. Randomized phase 2 study of GMI-1070 in SCD: Reduction in time to resolution of vaso-occlusive events and decreased opioid use. Blood. 2015;**125**(17):2656-2664. DOI: 10.1182/blood-2014-06-583351

[38] Ferreira de Matos C, Comont T, Castex MP, et al. Risk of vaso-occlusive episodes in patients with sickle cell disease exposed to systemic corticosteroids: A comprehensive review. Expert Review of Hematology. 2022;**15**(12):1045-1054. DOI: 10.1080/17474086.2022.2149488

[39] Joseph JJ, Abraham AA, Fitzhugh CD. When there is no match, the game is not over: Alternative donor options for hematopoietic stem cell transplantation in sickle cell disease. Seminars in Hematology. 2018;**55**:94-101. DOI: 10.1053/j.seminhematol.2018.04.013

[40] Shenoy S. Hematopoietic stem-cell transplantation for sickle cell disease: Current evidence and opinions. Therapeutic Advances in Hematology. 2013;**4**:335-344. DOI: 10.1177/2040620713483063

[41] Hanggi P, Makhro A, Gassmann M, Schmugge M, Goede JS, Speer O, et al. Red blood cells of sickle cell disease patients exhibit abnormally highabundanceofN-methylD-aspartat ereceptorsmediatingexcessivecalcium uptake. British Journal of Haematology. 2014;**167**:252-264. DOI: 10.1111/bjh.13028

[42] Telen MJ, Malik P, Vercellotti GM. Therapeutic strategies for sickle cell disease: Towards a multi-agent approach. Nature Reviews. Drug Discovery. 2019;**18**(2):139-158. DOI: 10.1038/s41573-018-0003-2

[43] Hoppe C, Jacob E, Styles L, Kuypers F, Larkin S, Vichinsky E. Simvastatin reduces vaso-occlusive pain in sickle cell anaemia: A pilot efficacy trial. British Journal of Haematology. 2017;**177**:620-629. DOI: 10.1111/bjh.14580

[44] Awojoodu AO, Keegan PM, Lane AR, Zhang Y, Lynch KR, Platt MO, et al. Acid sphingomyelinase is activated in sickle cell erythrocytes and contributes to inflammatory microparticle generation in SCD. Blood. 2014;**124**(12):1941-1950. DOI: 10.1182/blood-2014-01-543652

[45] David R, Yurdanur K, Selma U, Carlton D, Betty P, Banu K, et al. Double-blind, randomized study of canakinumab treatment in pediatric and young adult patients with sickle cell anemia. Blood. 2019;**134**:615-615. DOI: 10.1182/blood-2019-123355

[46] Adashi EY, Gruppuso PA, Cohen IG. CRISPR therapy of sickle cell disease: The dawning of the gene editing era. The American Journal of Medicine. 2024;**137**(5):390-392. DOI: 10.1016/j.amjmed.2023.12.018

Section 2

Diverse Contributions

Chapter 7

Neutropenia and Hematology Analyzer

Gulsum Feyza Turkes

Abstract

The automated hematology analyzer is used to analyze white blood cell (WBC) counts. WBC differentials (WBC-diff) can be measured using a diff-scattergram. This group includes neutrophil cells. Neutrophils, characterized by their multilobed nuclei and a diameter ranging from 12 to 15 μm, constitute about 50–70% of the leukocytes present in the bloodstream. They serve as the initial line of defense against infections in the body. Neutropenia is defined as a neutrophil count below the reference range. Neutropenia can be classified as either hematological causes or non-hematological causes. Non-hematologic causes include ethnicity, medical procedures, viral infections, autoimmune illnesses, sepsis, and congenital neutropenia. Hematological causes include myelodysplastic syndromes, acute leukemia, lymphoma, etc. The complete blood count CBC flags notify hematological analyzer operators of abnormal cell conditions, such as neutropenia. Neutropenia can manifest either independently or in conjunction with other flags. Neutropenia can be diagnosed through the utilization of peripheral blood smear tests. We can determine auto-verification rules with certain algorithms by performing a reflex test with these flags. Then, we can perform a peripheral smear analysis. The aim of this section is to explain the method that can provide early diagnosis to patients.

Keywords: hematology analyzer, WBC, neutropenia, auto-verification, flags in hematology analyzer, flagging interpretation, flag messages

1. Introduction

A complete blood count (CBC) is a hematology analysis that offers comprehensive details about all kinds of blood cells in the body. Developments in technology have enabled the use of automated instruments for measurement. It can be recognized as the primary diagnostic method for hematological diseases. Furthermore, it is a technique employed in the identification and monitoring of many different diseases. Leukocyte differential cell number is determined by creating a leukocyte differential distinction in the complete blood count, which in addition consists of the white blood cell (WBC) count, erythrocyte count, and platelet count. Due to the presence of suspicious factors during the CBC, the physician decides to perform additional tests and suggests a peripheral smear for the patient.

Previously, the examination of peripheral blood morphology was conducted using a microscope and a manual peripheral smear. Thanks to modern technology,

 IntechOpen

laboratory examination of peripheral smear morphology is currently possible with automated peripheral smear devices. Furthermore, doctors have the capability to digitally access and view morphological results on their personal computers. Within this digital setting, the physician not only assesses the morphologic findings but also expedites the diagnosis of patients. Subsequently, an accurate diagnosis can be acquired using flow cytometry using either a peripheral blood sample or a bone marrow sample.

With this digitalization in the field of hematology, it has become important to interpret the flag results on CBC devices. Developing algorithms and automatic peripheral smearing based on these flags can guide us in the early diagnosis of diseases. The neutropenia flag is one of them. It can be isolated or combined with other flags.

2. White blood cell count

White blood cells originate from pluripotent hematopoietic stem cells found in the bone marrow. Once they reach adulthood, they are then released into the peripheral bloodstream. Within the circulatory system, these cells can be classified into two primary groups: granulocytes and agranulocytes. Neutrophils, basophils, and eosinophils are categorized as granulocytes because they contain granules in their cytoplasm. Polymorphonuclear leukocytes (PMNL) are an alternative term for these cells. Lymphocytes and monocytes are categorized as agranulocytes because they lack granules in their cytoplasm. These cells are commonly known as mononuclear leukocytes. Leukocyte counts in modern automated complete blood count systems are calculated through the classification of cells based on their size and volume [1].

The electrical impedance approach, utilizing the Coulter principle, depends on the nonconductive characteristics of cells to ascertain their quantity and size. When quantifying WBC *via* this technique, the information can be shown in the form of a histogram. Cell size and concentration are measured [2].

Modern WBC analysis in analyzers often relies on laser light scattering techniques, such as those used in flow cytometry. WBCs are hydrodynamically focused through a flow cell and exposed to laser light, with the resulting scatter captured by photodetectors. The total WBC count is determined by the number of light interruptions. Forward scatter correlates with cell size, while 7° side scatter indicates internal cell complexity and 90° side scatter (lobularity) reflects cytoplasmic granularity [2].

The flow cytometry using a semiconductor laser counts and classifies cells by irradiating them with a 633 nm laser beam and analyzing their forward scattered light (FSC), side scattered light (SSC), and side fluorescent light (SFL). The intensity of the two types of scattered light (FSC and SSC) reflects cell surface structure, particle shape, nucleus form, refractive index, and reflectivity of the cells. In general, the FSC signal is stronger for larger cells, and the SSC signal becomes stronger as the intracellular structures become more complex. The intensity of the side fluorescent light mainly reflects the type and amount of nucleic acids and cell organelles. These three signals are used to differentiate and count white blood cells, nucleated red blood cells, reticulocytes, and platelets, and to detect abnormal cells and immature cells with the help of unique digital technology and algorithms [3]. The semiconductor laser flow cytometry approach involves conducting measurements over many channels. The WNR channel is utilized for the measurement of white blood cells (WBC). WBC quantification can be carried out by analyzing the

Age	Beckman Coulter DXH 900		Sysmex XN 3000	
	Female	Male	Female	Male
0 to <3 years	5.3–13.2	5.3–13.2	5.75–13.5	5.75–13.5
3 to <5 years	4.8–11.5	4.8–11.5	4.92–11.8	4.92–11.8
5 to <21 years	4.2–10.2	4.2–10.2	4.23–9.99	4.23–9.99

Table 1.
WBC reference range according to age group

forward scattered light and fluorescence intensity acquired from each cell using a two-dimensional scatter plot [4].

The reference ranges for WBC count in automated CBC devices, categorized by age, are displayed in **Table 1** [5, 6]. While the adult reference range for Turkey is 4.39–11.59 × 10^9/L, it was determined as 3.4–9.6 × 10^9/L in the Mayo Clinic Laboratory [7, 8].

Monoclonal antibodies and polyclonal antibodies are acceptable for validating measurement procedures. The term monoclonal antibody refers to one unique kind of antibody that is produced by a single lymphocyte cell. Monoclonal antibodies, which consist of antibody molecules that possess identical antigenic qualities, are very suitable for accurately measuring antigens. They find extensive use in various applications, including cell sorting. Typical blood consists of a combination of several antibody molecules generated by multiple B cells. Antibodies that consist of a mixture of various types of antibody molecules are referred to as polyclonal antibodies [9].

Many modern analyzers utilize fluorochrome-conjugated monoclonal antibodies, like those in flow cytometry, to enhance and broaden the differential cell count. The flow cytometry method utilizes fluorescent-labeled monoclonal antibodies (mAb). Monoclonal antibody (mAb) play a crucial role in diagnosing hematological illnesses and evaluating the immunophenotype for leukemia and lymphoma. The antigenic structures on the surface of human cells are referred to as clusters of differentiation (CD) to ensure standardized terminology. Through the selection of a suitable CD antibody, one can effectively and specifically mark the desired cells. Sysmex common antibodies, such as CD3, CD4, CD8, and CD34, are employed to identify T-cell subsets and immature cell populations [2].

2.1 White blood cell differential (WBC-Diff)

Differential counting of WBC types began approximately 120 years ago. Approximately 120 years ago, differential counting of leukocyte types began, marking a significant milestone in hematology. In 1891, Ehrlich developed a triacid stain for malarial parasites and differentiated neutrophilic cells, naming tissue cells with prominent granules' mast cells. Romanowsky, Giemsa, and Wright later modified the stain method to reveal subtle structures in nuclear chromatin and cytoplasmic granules. Gibson proposed the Gibson Chart, correlating leukocyte count with the severity of infection. Arneth classified neutrophils based on the number of lobes. Ehrlich's staining methods greatly advanced leukemia classification. Notably, Conan Doyle reported a case of leucocythemia in 1882, contributing to early awareness of blood disorders [10].

The history of blood counting and counting instruments is closely linked to the evolution of compound microscopes, which originated in the 1600s in the Netherlands. Microscopy-based cellular analysis began in the 1700s, with pioneers like von Leeuwenhoek. Paul Ehrlich played a crucial role in describing blood cell elements. Subsequently, Malassez and others utilized instruments like the hemocytometer for cell counts, and Neubauer refined manual enumeration techniques. In the twentieth century, centrifugation enabled the quantification of various blood fractions. Coulter's aperture impedance concept revolutionized hematology, leading to automated blood counting based on electric field suspension and cell separation. Multiparameter cell analyzers further advanced automated counting, culminating in modern hematology analyzers providing CBC [2].

Peripheral blood contains five distinct varieties of WBC-Diff. Differentiated leukocyte cells include monocytes, neutrophils, eosinophils, and basophils. In the peripheral bloodstream, neutrophils comprise the vast majority of WBC. Any variation in any of these factors has the possibility of impacting the WBC. Therefore, it is essential to carry out a WBC-diff analysis together with the WBC. White blood cell differential analysis can be performed either manually or with automated instruments. A manual WBC-diff analysis is conducted on a peripheral blood smear using microscopic imaging. For WBC-diff results, a total of 100 WBC are imaged and the different subtypes are quantified. WBC-diff analysis can be performed either manually or automatically. Automated imaging devices have replaced manual microscopy as the preferred method, although hand counting is still considered the most reliable. Clinicians can now use automated peripheral smear equipment to evaluate morphological data on their computers, thanks to modern technology. Automated imaging devices have replaced manual microscopy viewing with the advancement of technology, but manual counting is still considered the gold standard [11].

WBC enumeration and classification into different leukocyte types can be achieved through image analysis using proprietary software and algorithms. This method quantifies WBCs from a stained slide using a fixed volume of EDTA-anticoagulated blood. Stained cells are analyzed *via* automated digital microscopy employing an artificial neural network. The system allows manual review and sorting of unidentified cells before releasing results. These analysis systems show a strong correlation with other methods for the typical five-part differential, but there may be more variability in results for extended cell types, particularly immature granulocytes [2].

Automated CBC devices are also capable of conducting WBC-diff analysis. The 5-part or 7-part differentials are identified in the advanced hematology analyzer. An absolute quantity and a percentage are assigned to each cell type [12].

2.1.1 Neutrophile

Neutrophils are 12–15 μm in diameter and have multi-lobed nuclei. They are called polymorphonuclear neutrophils. Neutrophils comprise about 50–70% of circulating leukocytes and represent the body's initial line of defense. They are involved in the acute inflammatory response to bacterial infection and the removal of the bacteria by phagocytosis. Neutrophils, constituting 50–70% of circulating white blood cells, serve as the body's initial defense against infections. Primarily involved in the acute inflammatory response to bacterial infections, they remove bacteria through phagocytosis [13].

2.1.2 Neutrophil count

The result of the neutrophil count is of two types, like other WBC-diff. Both the absolute neutrophil count (NEU# - ANC) and the neutrophil percentage (NEU%) result should be included in the patient outcome report. While the ANC adult reference range for Turkey is 2.04–7.54 × 10^9/L, and the NEU% adult reference range is 40–74%, ANC was determined as 1.56–6.45 × 10^9/L in the Mayo Clinic Laboratory [7, 8]. ANC-validated reference ranges automated CBC devices according to age are shown in **Table 2**, while NEU%-validated reference ranges are shown in **Table 3** [5, 6].

2.1.3 Neutropenia

The term "neutropenia" is used to describe a reduction in blood neutrophil count below the reference range in CBC devices. The international consensus group for hematology review recommends a threshold value of 1 × 10^9/L for neutropenia in peripheral smear while the French Speaking Cellular Hematology Group (GFCH) recommends 1.5 × 10^9/L [14, 15].

Bone marrow hypoplasia-associated neutropenia may occur as either primary or secondary. The primary causes are rarely observed. The primary causes include leukocyte adhesion deficiency, Chediak-Higashi syndrome, hyper-IgE syndrome, recurrent infection syndrome, and chronic granulomatous illness. Secondary causes are prevalent and encompass cytotoxic medications, aplastic anemia, leukemia, drug hypersensitivity responses, and infections [16].

Apart from primary and secondary causes, neutropenia can be divided into two groups: hematological diseases and non-hematological conditions [14].

Non-hematologic causes: possible causes include ethnic factors, medical procedures, viral infections, autoimmune disorders, sepsis or congenital neutropenia.

10^9/L	**Beckman Coulter DXH 900**		**Sysmex XN 3000**	
Age	**Female**	**Male**	**Female**	**Male**
0 to <1 years	0.9–4.6	0.9–4.6	0.69–5.82	0.69–5.82
1 to <21 years	1.5–6.4	1.5–6.4	1.45–6.75	1.45–6.75

Table 2.
Absolute neutrophil count reference range.

%	**Beckman Coulter DXH 900**		**Sysmex XN 3000**	
Age	**Female**	**Male**	**Female**	**Male**
0 to <1 years	9.2–45.3	9.2–45.3	8.7–57.9	8.7–57.9
1 to <5 years	17.6–68.1	17.6–68.1	18.6–68.6	18.6–68.6
5 to <15 years	29.7–68.6	29.7–68.6	28.9–67.9	28.9–67.9
15 to <21 years	42.8–75.1	41.3–76.1	39.6–73.9	42.8–75.1

Table 3.
Neutrophil percentage reference range.

Congenital neutropenia encompasses a group of neutropenic disorders that can be persistent or intermittent, severe (<0.5 10^9/L) or mild (between 0.5 and 1.5 10^9/L), and can also affect other organ systems such as the pancreas, central nervous system, heart, muscles, and skin. Congenital neutropenia has two primary groups: those without extra-hematopoietic symptoms and those with. No additional organs are involved in congenital neutropenia without extra-hematopoietic symptoms. This category includes ELANE (ELA2), extracellular G-CSF receptor abnormalities, GFI1-associated neutropenia, and WAS gene mutation-induced lifelong congenital neutropenia. Congenital neutropenia with extra-hematopoietic symptoms involves various organs. Kostmann disease, HAX1 mutations, Shwachman-Diamond syndrome, G6PC3 mutations, Cohen syndrome, Poikiloderma, Clericuzio type, Barth syndrome, AP14 deficiency, and Hermansky Pudlak syndrome type 2 are congenital neutropenia diseases with extra-hematopoietic manifestations [17].

During viral infections, the automated hematology analyzer frequently identifies an "Atypical Lymphocytes" flag. This is typically caused by the presence of activated lymphocytes or the actual mononucleosis syndrome. Severe sepsis can manifest as a condition characterized by low levels of neutrophils and platelets, together with an indication of an abnormal increase in immature white blood cells, which warrants a study of a peripheral blood smear. In cases of autoimmune or iatrogenic neutropenia, the condition often involves a decrease in neutrophil count, and examining a blood smear has minimal influence on the treatment of the patient [14].

Hematological causes: possible causes include acute leukemia (AL), myelodysplastic syndromes (MDS), lymphoma malignancies, hairy cell leukemia (HCL), large granular lymphocytic leukemia (LGL) acute monoblastic leukemia (AML-M5a), acute erythroid leukemia (AML-M6), AML with myelodysplasia-related changes, myelodysplastic syndrome—refractory anemia with excess blasts (RAEB 2), acute myeloblastic leukemia without maturation (M1), acute promyelocytic leukemia (APL), multiple myelome (MM), B-cell lymphobhlastic leukemia (B-ALL), Pelger-Huet anomaly-2, etc. [14, 18, 19].

2.1.4 Flags in hematology analyzers

Auto-verification is the computer-based interpretation of clinical biochemistry analysis results used within the framework of certain rules algorithm determination or machine learning [20]. By reducing manual interpretation time, it prevents extra effort and unintentional errors made in thousands of patients. By focusing on truly problematic cases, staff can interpret the results more accurately [21].

Auto-verification rules include device flags, reference range, analytical measurement range, critical value, mathematical or logical error, clot, delta check, etc. Algorithms determined within the framework of these rules should be determined and verified using the Clinical and Laboratory Standards Institute (CLSI) guideline, AUTO10-A (Autoverification of Clinical Laboratory Test Results) and CLSI guideline, AUTO15-ED1:2019 (Autoverification of Medical Laboratory Results for Specific Disciplines) [18].

In the field of hematology, the term "flag" refers to signals that are displayed to operators to indicate the presence of abnormal cell conditions. The presence of abnormalities in the CBC can offer valuable flags for doing further examinations on patients. Neutropenia is a condition that falls within this category. Peripheral smear testing is primarily indicated for the diagnosis of neutropenia. Neutropenia can occur

Flags	Meaning
<	Low the analytical measurement range
>	High the analytical measurement range
L	Low the reference range
H	High the reference range
Abn. WBC Scattergram	Abnormal WBC Scattergram
Pancytopenia	Low WBC-Diff cells
Neutropenia	Low neutrophil count
Lymphopenia	Low lymphocyte count
Lymphocytosis	High lymphocyte count
Monocytosis	High monocyte count
Basophilia	High basophil count
Leukocytopenia	Low leukocyte count
NRBC present	High nucleated RBC count
IG present	Increased immature granulocyte
Blasts/Abn Lympho?	Possibility that blasts are present/ Possibility of abnormal lymphocytes
Blasts?	Possibility that blasts are present
Abn Lympho?	Possibility of abnormal lymphocytes
Left Shift?	Possibility of left shift
Atypical lympho?	Possibility of atypical lymphocytes
Variant Lymphs?	Possibility of variant lymphocytes

Table 4.
Flags in hematology analyzers for WBC and WBC-diff analysis

either on its own or in conjunction with other flags abnormal cells or morphological abnormalities associated with hematological disorders are rarely observed in peripheral blood smear results when isolated neutropenia is present. Nevertheless, peripheral smear results can be significant when there are additional flags of neutropenia [14].

There are many flags regarding WBC analysis that may accompany neutropenia in automated CBC analyzers. The flags are listed in **Table 4**.

2.1.5 Cases and flags

The following sample cases include the analysis results observed at the time of first admission to the hospital.

2.1.5.1 Acute promyelocytic leukemia (APL)

CBC flags: Abn. WBC scattergram, Blasts?, Abn Lymph/blast?, Immature Gran?, basophilia, leukocytosis, anemia, thrombocytopenia, L for ANC, L for NEU%, H for WBC, L for eosinophil, and H for basophil.

Peripheral blood morphology examination: Low segmented neutrophil count, low lymphocyte count, and blasts are present [18].

2.1.5.2 Multiple myeloma (MM)

CBC flags: *Pancytopenia*, Blasts?, Abn Lymph/blast?, Atypical Lymph?, L for ANC, L for NEU%, L for WBC, L for eosinophil, L for eosinophil%, H for lymphocyte%, and H for monocyte%.

Peripheral blood morphology examination: Low segmented neutrophil count, high lymphocyte count, low monocyte count, and plasma cells are present [18].

2.1.5.3 B-cell lymphoblastic leukemia (B-ALL)

CBC flags: Blasts?, Abn Lymph/blast?, Immature Gran?, L for ANC, L for NEU%, L for monocyte, L for monocyte%, H for eosinophil, and H for eosinophil%.

Peripheral blood morphology examination: *Low segmented neutrophil count*, low monocyte count, high eosinophil count, and myelocytes is present. Blasts and abnormal lymphocytes are present [18].

2.1.5.4 B-cell lymphoblastic leukemia (B-ALL)

CBC flags: Abn. WBC scattergram, Abn Lymph/blast?, Immature Gran?, lymphocytosis, *neutropenia*, leukocytosis, anemia, thrombocytopenia, L for ANC, L for NEU%, L for eosinophil, L for eosinophil%, H for WBC, H for lymphocyte, and L for monocyte%.

Peripheral blood morphology examination: Low segmented neutrophil count, blasts are present [18].

2.1.5.5 Mantle cell lymphoma (MCL)

CBC flags: Abn. WBC scattergram, Abn Lymph/blast?, Lymphocytosis, L for ANC, L for NEU%, H for WBC, H for lymphocyte, and H for lymphocyte%.

Peripheral blood morphology examination: *Low segmented neutrophil count*, low monocyte count, high lymphocyte count, blasts, reactive lymphocytes, and abnormal lymphocytes are present [18].

2.1.5.6 Pelger–Huët anomaly

CBC flags: *Pancytopenia*, lymphopenia, leukocytopenia, anemia, thrombocytopenia, L for ANC, H for NEU%, L for WBC, L for lymphocyte, L for monocyte, L for eosinophil, and L for eosinophil%.

Peripheral blood morphology examination: low segmented neutrophil count, high band neutrophil count, low monocyte count, and metamyelocytes are present [18].

2.1.5.7 Acute monoblastic leukemia (AML-M5a)

CBC flags: *Neutropenia,* monocytosis, blasts?, anemia, trombocytopenia.

Peripheral blood morphology examination: Low segmented neutrophil count, blasts, and monoblasts are present [19].

2.1.5.8 Acute erythroid leukemia (AML-M6)

CBC flags: *Neutropenia,* leukocytopenia, NRBC present, blasts?, anisocytosis, macrocytosis, anemia, fragments?

Peripheral blood morphology examination: Low segmented neutrophil count, myeloblasts, and NRBC are present [19].

2.1.5.9 AML with myelodysplasia-related changes

CBC flags: *Neutropenia*, Blasts?, anisocytosis, and anemia.

Peripheral blood morphology examination: Low segmented neutrophil count, myeloblasts , and NRBC is present [19].

2.1.5.10 Myelodysplastic syndrome—refractory anemia with excess blasts (RAEB-2)

CBC flags: *Neutropenia,* lymphopenia, leukocytopenia, NRBC present, blasts?, anisocytosis, macrocytosis, fragments?, PLT Abn distribution?, and thrombocytopenia.

Peripheral blood morphology examination: Low segmented neutrophil count, myeloblast , and NRBC is present [19].

2.1.5.11 Acute myeloid leukemia (AML-M0)

CBC flags: variant lymphs?, blasts?, NRBC present, L for ANC, L for NEU%, L for monocyte, L for monocyte%, and H for lymphocyte%.

Peripheral blood morphology examination: low segmented neutrophil count, blasts are present, and high lymphocyte count [22].

2.1.5.12 MDS with monosomy 7 presenting as aplastic anemia

CBC flags: NRBC present, L for ANC.

Peripheral blood morphology examination: NRBC and Pelger-Huët cells are present [22].

2.1.5.13 T-cell large granular lymphocyte leukemia

CBC flags: Variant lymphs?, NRBC present, L for ANC, L for NEU%, L for monocyte, H for lymphocyte, H for lymphocyte%, L for monocyte%, L for eosinophil%, L for basophil%

Peripheral blood morphology examination: low segmented neutrophil count, large granular lymphocytes, smudge cells, and some big platelets are present [22].

In many cases, such as the ones listed above, a conclusive diagnosis is established by further tests after the analysis of the CBC test, which serves as the initial screening examination. Upon analyzing the CBC results, the hemato-oncologist may recommend additional tests if they are judged appropriate. Nevertheless, contemporary algorithms have been devised as a substitute for this prolonged approach [23]. Most tests are added by automated analyzers, using algorithms devised by laboratory professionals. This process is known as "reflex testing" [24]. The reflex test allows for the performance of a peripheral smear test using the same sample following automated hematological analysis, which serves as the initial screening procedure. Hence, it is crucial to study and interpret the flag data obtained from the hematological analyzer. When neutropenia is present, the time it takes to get results known as the turnaround time (TAT) is reduced by using the peripheral smear test as a reflex test [23].

3. Conclusion

Complete blood count devices are used primarily to screen for hematology patients. Since automated peripheral smear devices have been developed, they can be considered as a screening test. Since additional diseases, especially malignancy, are observed in patients with neutropenia report results, neutropenia should be included in the auto-verification rules. In these patients, peripheral smear analysis should first be performed from the same sample with the reflex test rule. In this way, the advantage of more accurate and earlier diagnosis can be obtained for patients.

Conflict of interest

The author declares no conflict of interest.

Acronyms and abbreviations

CBC	complete blood cell
WBC	white blood cell
WBC-Diff	white blood cell differential
PMNL	polymorphonuclear leukocytes
EDTA	Etilendiamin tetraasetik asit
ANC	absolute neutrophil count
NEU%	neutrophil percentage
GFCH	the French Speaking Cellular Hematology Group
CLSI	Clinical and Laboratory Standards Institute
RBC	red blood cell

Author details

Gulsum Feyza Turkes[1,2]

1 Department of Medical Biochemistry, Medicine Faculty, Ankara University, Ankara, Turkey

2 Department of Medical Biochemistry, Graduate School of Health Sciences, Gazi University, Ankara, Turkey

*Address all correspondence to: gfeyzaa90@gmail.com

References

[1] Konukoğlu D. Kan Hastalıklarına Biyokimyasal ve Laboratuvar Yaklaşım. 1st ed. Istanbul: Nobel Tıp Kitabevleri Ltd Şti; 2022. p. 489

[2] Rifai N. Tietz Textbook of Laboratory Medicine. 7th ed. Health Science. United States: Elsevier; 2022. p. 1584

[3] Matsushita H, Tanaka Y, Sakairi K, et al. XN-Series Clinical Case Report. Vol. 2. Japan: Sysmex Corporation Scientific Affairs; 2012

[4] Sysmex Corporation Scientific Affairs. Germany: Sysmex Corporation; 2018. pp. 1-41

[5] Tahmasebi H, Higgins V, Kathryn Bohn M, et al. CALIPER hematology reference standards (I): Improving laboratory test interpretation in children (Beckman Coulter DxH 900–Core Laboratory Hematology System). American Journal of Clinical Pathology. 2020;**154**:330-341. DOI: 10.1093/ajcp/aqaa059

[6] Bohn MK, Higgins V, Tahmasebi H, et al. Complex biological patterns of hematology parameters in childhood necessitating age- and sex-specific reference intervals for evidence-based clinical interpretation. International Journal of Laboratory Hematology. 2020;**42**:750-760. DOI: 10.1111/ijlh.13306

[7] Ozarda Y, Ichihara K, Bakan E, et al. A nationwide multicentre study in Turkey for establishing reference intervals of haematological parameters with novel use of a panel of whole blood. Biochemia Medica (Zagreb). 15 Jun 2017;**27**(2):350-377. DOI: 10.11613/BM.2017.038

[8] Mayo Clinic Lab. CBC – Overview: Complete blood cell count (CBC) with differential, Blood. 2024. Available from: https://www.mayocliniclabs.com/test-catalog/overview/9109#Clinical-and-Interpretive [Accessed January 04, 2024]

[9] Sysmex. Easy to Understand XN Series Measuring Principles. Japan: Sysmex Corporation Scientific Affairs; 2016

[10] Tatsumi N, Pierre RV. Automated image processing past, present, and future of blood cell morphology identification. Clinics in Laboratory Medicine. Mar 2022;**22**(1):299-315. DOI: 10.1016/s0272-2712(03)00076-3

[11] Yoon S, Hur M, Lee GH, Nam M, Kim H. How reproducible is the data from sysmex DI-60 in leukopenic samples? Diagnostics (Basel). 23 Nov 2021;**11**(12):2173. DOI: 10.3390/diagnostics11122173

[12] Chhabra G. Automated hematology analyzers: Recent trends and applications. Journal of Lab Physicians. 2018;**10**:15-16. DOI: 10.4103/JLP.JLP_124_17

[13] Tigner A, Ibrahim SA, Murray IV. Histology, White Blood Cell. [Updated 2022 Nov 14]. In: StatPearls [Internet]. Treasure Island (FL): StatPearls Publishing; Jan 2024. Available from: https://www.ncbi.nlm.nih.gov/books/NBK563148/ [Accessed: January 01, 2024]

[14] Ronez E, Geara C, Coito S, et al. Usefulness of thresholds for smear review of neutropenic samples analyzed with a Sysmex XN-10 analyzer. Scandinavian Journal of Clinical and Laboratory Investigation. 2017;77:406-409. DOI: 10.1080/00365513.2017.1334129

[15] Geneviève F, Mercier-Bataille D, Wagner-Ballon O, et al. Smear

microscopy revision: Propositions by the GFHC. Feuillets de Biologie (Vol LVI N° 317) Hematology. 2014

[16] Justiz Vaillant AA, Zito PM. Neutropenia. [Updated 2022 Aug 25]. In: StatPearls [Internet]. Treasure Island (FL): StatPearls Publishing; Jan 2024. Available from: https://www.ncbi.nlm.nih.gov/books/NBK507702/ [Accessed: January 05, 2024]

[17] Donadieu J, Fenneteau O, Beaupain B, et al. Congenital neutropenia: Diagnosis, molecular bases and patient management. Orphanet Journal of Rare Disease. 2011;**6**:26. DOI: 10.1186/1750-1172-6-26

[18] Mindray. Hemacase Clinical Case Booklet. Vol. 1. Shenzen: Shenzhen Mindray Bio-Medical Electronics Co., Ltd; 2023

[19] Matsushita H, Tanaka Y, Sakairi K, et al. XN-Series Clinical Case Report. 1st ed. Vol. 1. Japan: Sysmex Corporation Scientific Affairs; 2011

[20] Harrison JH, Gilbertson JR, Hanna MG, et al. Introduction to artificial intelligence and machine learning for pathology. Archives of Pathology & Laboratory Medicine. 2021;**145**:1228-1254. DOI: 10.5858/arpa.2020-0541-CP

[21] Krasowski MD, Davis SR, Drees D, et al. Autoverification in a core clinical chemistry laboratory at an academic medical center. Journal of Pathology Informatics. 28 Mar 2014;**5**(1):13. DOI: 10.4103/2153-3539.129450

[22] Simon-Lopez R, Solenthaler M, Jeanneret C, Capel J, Rusanova E, et al. UniCel DxH Series Case Book – The Process of CBC-diff Analysis in the Modern Hematology. Beckman Coulter; 2013

[23] Roland K, Yakimec J, Markin T, et al. Customized middleware experience in a tertiary care hospital hematology laboratory. Journal of Pathology Informatics. 2022;**13**:100143. DOI: 10.1016/j.jpi.2022.100143

[24] Srivastava R, Bartlett WA, Kennedy IM, et al. Reflex and reflective testing: Efficiency and effectiveness of adding on laboratory tests. Annals of Clinical Biochemistry. 2010;**47**:223-227. DOI: 10.1258/acb.2010.009282

Chapter 8

The Role of Inherited Coagulopathies in the Development of Primary and Secondary Postpartum Hemorrhage

Jolana Schmiedl and Giancarlo Castaman

Abstract

Postpartum hemorrhage (PPH) remains the leading cause of maternal death worldwide, despite advances in diagnostic and management of massive bleeding in recent decades. It accounts for 25 percent of maternal deaths annually. Nearly 14 million women experience PPH each year, leading to 280,000 deaths globally [World PPH Summit 2023, Dubai]. PPH is preventable and requires increased attention to inherited causes of massive bleeding, which are often underestimated and lead to late diagnosis. The recent report from the Centers for Disease Control and Prevention (CDC) emphasizes the urgent need for action in low- and middle-income countries. However, high-income countries are also impacted by global movements that may negatively affect trends in maternal deaths. This chapter addresses the role of different coagulation factors in developing primary and secondary PPH, the importance of a multidisciplinary approach, and the significance of treatment protocols in obstetric settings. Additionally, we discuss the current guidelines for managing PPH and how recent developments in the diagnosis and treatment of inherited bleeding disorders could influence the management of PPH.

Keywords: blood loss, coagulation factors, late diagnostic, treatment algorithm, multidisciplinary approach

1. Introduction

Hemorrhage at parturition is the leading cause of maternal death worldwide [1]. Bleeding complications during and after delivery can lead to death within hours if women are left unattended. In 2020, there was almost one death every 2 minutes among women, and most of these deaths are preventable [2], with low and lower-middle-income countries being the most affected. Despite a global drop of 34% in maternal mortality between 2000 and 2020, the rate is still unacceptably high at 223 per 100,000 live births. In 2020, Sub-Saharan Africa and Southern Asia accounted for close to 87 percent of all estimated global maternal deaths, with Sub-Saharan Africa alone contributing to around 70 percent and Southern Asia to 16 percent of the world's maternal deaths. In the USA, the maternal mortality rate decreased to 22.3 deaths per 100,000 live births in 2022, compared with 32.9 in 2021 [3]. However, United Nations data released in early 2023 showed a reduction in maternal mortality from 2016 to 2020 in 133 countries while also indicating an increase in 17 countries, mainly in Latin America, the Caribbean, some countries in Europe, North America, and Sub-Saharan Africa [1]. Although the significant burden of maternal death persists in low and low-middle-income countries (LMICs), recent data from high-income countries (HICs) suggests that marginalized, neglected, racialized, and immigrant groups face significantly increased risks. In certain marginalized groups in HICs, particularly in the USA, maternal mortality rates exceed those in LMICs [4]. In addition, the age of women who give birth in developed countries has increased, which has led to an increased risk of PPH due to repeated cesarean deliveries in this group [5].

The World Health Organization (WHO) is acting against the current trend in maternal mortality with its first roadmap to tackle PPH, which is defined as excessive bleeding after birth. PPH affects millions of women and is the world's leading cause of maternal death [6].

Bleeding complications during and after delivery are commonly caused by obstetrical complications such as atonic uterus (80%) and complications due to trauma events on the uterus (20%). While inherited bleeding disorders represent only nearly 1% of bleeding complications during and postpartum, they can lead to difficult-to-manage bleeding. Congenital bleeding disorders are often overlooked, as they are diagnosed late and are not the focus of gynecologists and obstetricians [7, 8]. The most common cause of PPH, apart from obstetric complications, infection, eclampsia, and unsafe delivery, is missing or malfunctioning coagulation factors. The diagnostic focus in PPH requires substantial attention, in particular to von Willebrand factor (vWF), fibrinogen, factor XIII (F XIII), and factor XI (FXI), but carriers for hemophilia A and B are of utmost importance according to the variability of clinical and laboratory phenotypes.

2. Coagulopathies and postpartum hemorrhage

2.1 Postpartum hemorrhage: Definition

PPH is a rare but potentially life-threatening condition. Based on a meta-analysis of 31 studies, its global prevalence is estimated between 6 and 10%, depending on the type of study. While the observational studies showed a prevalence close to 6 percent, the clinical randomized trials reveal a prevalence near 14 percent; a prevalence of 3 percent was observed during vaginal delivery. The recently published study from a cohort in China showed a higher incidence in nulliparous compared to multi-parous, 2.1 and 1.7 percent, respectively [9]. WHO defined the following risk factors for PPH: multiple pregnancies in general, multiple pregnancies—more than 5, coagulopathy, including both congenital and acquired coagulopathy, age over 30, anomalous placenta attachment, anemia, multiple pregnancies, and macrosomia [10].

In 2017, the American College of Obstetricians and Gynecologists (ACOG) defined postpartum hemorrhage (PPH) as greater than 500 mL of estimated blood loss during vaginal delivery or greater than 1000 mL of estimated blood loss during cesarean section. Due to challenges in accurately estimating blood loss, ACOG updated the definition to include cumulative blood loss greater than 1000 mL accompanied by signs of hypovolemia within 24 hours of delivery, regardless of the route of delivery. Primary PPH typically occurs within 1 day of giving birth, while secondary PPH can occur from 24 hours up to 12 weeks postpartum [11]. The traditional definition of primary PPH, used by the Royal College of Obstetricians and Gynecologists (RCOG), is blood loss of 500 mL or more from the genital tract following delivery. RCOG also distinguishes between minor PPH, with blood loss of 500–1000 mL, and major PPH, with blood loss of more than 1000 mL, which can be further categorized as moderate (1000–2000 mL) or severe (more than 2000 mL) blood loss. Several publications for gynecologists, obstetricians, family physicians, and nurses refer to the 4 T causes of PPH, while others list primary and secondary causes. Categorizing the causes of PPH should help ensure proportional attention to each potential cause in order to offer proper treatment for affected women. Inherited bleeding disorders are also mentioned, but several surveys and observational studies have shown delayed diagnosis of such disorders in women with abnormal bleeding, with some cases diagnosed during primary or secondary PPH [7, 8]. Delays in diagnosis are likely due to a lack of interdisciplinary approach, limited access to healthcare facilities in the developing world, insufficient information about family history of PPH and bleeding disorders, a lack of diagnostic tools, restricted access to appropriate treatment options, as well as religious and cultural factors. In addition to education and awareness campaigns, advancements in diagnostics and recommendations for appropriate treatment could facilitate earlier diagnosis and more effective treatment of PPH.

Primary causes (4 T): Tonus (reduced or minimal tone in the uterus), Trauma (uterus laceration, uterine inversion, placenta retention, and vaginal trauma), Tissue (abnormal placentation), and Thrombin (decreased thrombin generation due to coagulopathy).

Secondary causes: Retained products of conception, infection, subinvolution of the placental site, and inherited bleeding disorders.

2.2 Changes in the coagulation factors during pregnancy and postpartum

Changes in coagulation are usually observed during pregnancy, typically to produce a "para-physiologic" pro-thrombotic state to reduce the risk of bleeding. Women with inherited bleeding disorders face complexity in diagnostic and treatment recommendations due to these changes. Hormonal changes, especially estradiol-induced triglyceride alteration, result in increased levels of coagulation factors like VII, VIII, X, I (fibrinogen), and von Willebrand factor in healthy women during pregnancy, but often also in women with mild deficiencies of these factors prior to pregnancy. Additionally, the inhibition of protein S and fibrinolytic activity contributes to a shift toward low-grade coagulant activity. Despite these changes, the concentration of fibronectin remains unaffected before and during pregnancy, indicating no endothelial damage.

The physiological changes during pregnancy lead to hypercoagulation, providing protection from excessive blood loss during delivery. However, the pattern described shifts after delivery, with levels of coagulation factors and protein S declining within 1–3 weeks postpartum and returning to baseline after 5–12 weeks. The mode of delivery can impact the time it takes for levels to normalize. Similarly, changes in coagulation factor levels are expected also in women with inherited bleeding disorders, especially in those with mild and moderate forms, whose symptoms may have been overlooked before pregnancy.

Notably, hormonal therapy (HT) can mask bleeding symptoms in mild and moderate forms of von Willebrand disease (VWD) and carriers of Hemophilia A and B, posing risks of primary and secondary postpartum hemorrhage (PPH) if not properly diagnosed. Women with VWD and rare bleeding disorders (RBD) experience more bleeding complications during pregnancy compared to normal control groups. In a survey, 62 percent of gynecologists would refer women with heavy menstrual bleeding, a common symptom of VWD, to a hematologist only after failed HT for more than 1 to 5 years [7].

Von Willebrand factor (vWF) is the largest glycoprotein found in human plasma. VWF is synthesized in endothelial cells and megakaryocytes. VWF plays an essential role in the primary and secondary hemostasis. Its main function is mediating the adhesion of platelets to the site of vessel injury by interacting with a specific platelet surface receptor (GpIb) and contributing to platelet aggregation together with fibrinogen by binding to a second platelet receptor (GpIIb/IIIa). In addition, vWF carries 80 percent of FVIII protein in circulation, protecting it from proteolysis. The deficiency of vWF results in von Willebrand disease (VWD), an autosomal inherited bleeding disorder mainly manifested as mucocutaneous bleeding and, in more severe cases, in muscles, soft tissues, and joints. VWD equally affects males and females, although the diagnosis in females is usually delayed as diverse intensity of physiological bleeding in women is perceived as normal, and women would probably first consult gynecologists, family doctors, or pediatricians, but not hematologists. Recently published data suggested that 20–40 years of age is the time for diagnosing in women, while in men, it is approximately 6 years earlier [8, 12]. Depending on the type of mutation, the deficiency can be quantitative—VWD Type 1 and Type 3, or qualitative—VWD Type 2. The qualitative deficiency with reduced platelet-depended function accompanied by the lack of high and intermediate molecular weight VWF multimers is classified as Type 2A VWD, and Type 2B is due to VWF variants with enhanced affinity for platelets receptor GPlb, while Type 2 M is characterized by a reduced platelet-dependent function, but with the presence of high and intermediate molecular weight VWF multimers. Type 2 N is a qualitative variant with a significantly reduced affinity to factor VIII. Type 1 is the most prevalent type (55–70 percent of cases) and presents a relative reduction of VWF concentration and activity. Type 2 occurs in 15–20 percent of diagnosed patients with VWD while type 3 is the most severe type, characterized by the complete absence of WVF, with a prevalence of 1–3 percent of diagnosed individuals. Gestation influences the level of VWF in healthy women with VWF antigen level raised about 2–3 times, compared to levels before pregnancy. These levels return to non-pregnant values within 8–12 weeks postpartum.

Historical reports have shown that women with VWD are at a higher risk of developing primary and secondary PPH compared to healthy population, with rates of 29% versus 3–5%. Similarly, a published study by Kirtava et al. reported a 59% risk of PPH in women with VWD compared to 21% in those without VWD [13]. Data from the National Perinatal Information System in Slovenia also indicated a greater likelihood of developing primary PPH for women with VWD compared to those without; 7.7 and 2.2 percent, respectively (OR 3.7; 95% CI: 0.9–15.8) and a higher likelihood of requiring transfusion 24 hours after delivery (OR 16.3; 95% [14].

Close monitoring of FVIII/VWF changes is essential during pregnancy, delivery, and postpartum for individuals with Type 1 and Type 2 VWD, as different causative *VWF* variants can differently affect their changes. Levels of FVIII and VWF progressively increase during pregnancy and may reach normal ranges in Type 1 VWD.

However, baseline levels need careful monitoring, as women with VWF levels <20 IU/dL before pregnancy often do not experience a clinically meaningful increase in VWF during pregnancy. This is likely due to the presence of DNA variants associated with increased clearance of VWF and decreased synthesis and secretion. The variability in possible carriers of heterozygotes and heterogeneity in DNA variants underscores the importance of genetic testing, ideally before pregnancy and/or careful monitoring during pregnancy, especially in the third trimester, during delivery if treatment is used, and postpartum. In addition, the atonic uterus and other obstetric complications could contribute to an increased risk of PPH [15].

In Type 2A VWD, high molecular weight multimers do not usually appear during pregnancy, and low VWF:RCo levels still remain, although an increase in FVIII and VWF:Ag is typically observed. Type 2 B VWD is characterized by the enhanced affinity of VWF to the platelet's receptor glycoprotein Ib-alpha, resulting in variable thrombocytopenia. This pattern can be amplified during pregnancy, with severe thrombocytopenia sometimes being observed. Heterogeneity in DNA variants can result in varying platelet counts, so women with Type 2 B VWD should be monitored for their platelet count [16].

For Type 2 M VWD, FVIII, and VWF, Ag levels usually reach normal ranges during pregnancy, while VWF:RCo does generally not reach levels nearly to 50 IU/dl. Changes in the level of FVIII, VWF:Ag and VWF:RCo in Type 2 N commonly result in normal ranges during pregnancy, in homozygote as well as in heterozygote mutation R845Q; however, the levels are reduced in homozygotes soon after delivery [17].

Type 3 is the most severe form of von Willebrand disease (VWD), and it is autosomal recessive, unlike most of the other variants. Due to its pathophysiology, no changes in the levels of factor VIII (FVIII) and von Willebrand factor (VWF) are expected during pregnancy. This means that prophylaxis with replacement products during pregnancy and after childbirth is typically required, just as it is in most cases before pregnancy [15, 18].

Because VWD is complex and the DNA analysis is not routinely available, it is important to carefully monitor women with VWD during pregnancy. If treatment with desmopressin or replacement products is used, accurate monitoring in the first days after parturition is similarly required. It is essential to involve a multidisciplinary team, including hematologists and gynecologists/obstetrics to plan delivery modalities to prevent bleeding complications in pregnant women. Additionally, seeking advice from hematologists at the first signs of bleeding complications can be beneficial, as even mild forms of VWD affected by obstetric complications could lead to severe blood loss during and after delivery.

FVIII and FIX in hemophilia carriers: Hemophilia A and B are X-linked bleeding disorders characterized by a deficiency of coagulation factor FVIII and FIX, resulting in bleeding symptoms mainly in males. While 80 percent of hemophilia carriers have sufficient coagulation factor levels for normal blood clotting, some individuals may remain with low factor levels by the end of pregnancy, putting them at increased risk of bleeding complications during and after childbirth. A systematic literature review found that the incidence of postpartum hemorrhage (PPH) in hemophilia carriers without prophylaxis was 77%, while it was 44% in women with prophylaxis in individual cases and about 20% in cohort data, regardless of prophylaxis [19].

The variability of clotting factor levels in carriers has been observed by several researchers, with carriers generally having factor levels close to half of non-carriers. During pregnancy, FVIII levels can increase by 2 or 3-fold, while FIX levels increase only slightly. In a survey of 225 carriers conducted by Plug et al., the mean clotting factor level in carriers was 0.60 (0.05–2.1) IU/mL, compared to 1.02 (0.45–3.28) IU/mL in 143 non-carriers. Similarly, findings published by Stoof et al. showed that factor levels in carriers of hemophilia A and B before pregnancy were 0.65 (0.36–1.15) and 0.67 (0.22–0.93), respectively. In the mentioned study population, out of 95 hemophilia A carriers, 33 (35%) developed PPH, with 5 (5.3%) experiencing blood loss ≥1000 mL. Among 19 hemophilia B carriers, 9 (47%) experienced PPH, and 2 (10.5%) had blood loss of ≥1000 mL. Interestingly, the results of this study showed an increased risk of PPH in women who received prophylactic treatment compared to deliveries without prophylaxis, with an odds ratio of 3.2 (95% CI, 0.9–11.0). The authors also found that a higher incidence of PPH was noted in women with factor levels at the third trimester <0.20 IU/mL. These findings indicate the importance of closely monitoring the levels of coagulation factors in carriers during pregnancy, especially in the third trimester and close to delivery, to mitigate the risk of PPH and to adopt the appropriate anti-hemorrhagic prophylaxis [20, 21].

Factor XI (FXI) is a unique coagulation factor, consisting of identical subunits that form a dimer. It was previously referred to as plasma thromboplastin antecedent (PTA), and its deficiency is known as Rosenthal syndrome or hemophilia C. FXI plays a role in the intrinsic coagulation pathway, being activated by thrombin, FVIIa, and tissue factor at the site of injury. Once activated, FXI (FXIa) then activates FIX to form FIXa, supporting further thrombin generation [22].

In addition to its role in the coagulation cascade, FXI may also be involved in the kallikrein–kinin system, a group of proteins associated with host defense and homeostasis. Researchers attribute the unique structure and role of FXI to evolutionary influences across different species [22]. Unlike FVIII and FIX deficiencies, FXI deficiency is not linked to the X chromosome and typically occurs as an autosomal recessive or dominant trait.

The prevalence of FXI deficiency varies, ranging from 0 in 1,000,000 in countries with limited resources and inadequate diagnostics, to 55–85/million in the UK, according to the World Federation of Hemophilia's 2020 report. A study by Bauduer et al. in the French Basque country reported the highest prevalence at 246.2 in 1,000,000, noting that differences in prevalence can be explained by the variety of mutations associated with FXI deficiency. Notably, patients in Nantes also demonstrated a high prevalence of the condition.

In both England and among Ashkenazi Jews, women with FXI deficiency typically experience heavy menstrual bleeding. However, this does not necessarily indicate a predictive sign for the risk of postpartum hemorrhage (PPH). In low-resource countries, patients with FXI deficiency may go undiagnosed due to mild symptoms or be misdiagnosed with another clotting disorder. Severe FXI deficiency is defined as having a factor activity level of 15 percent or less, and these patients are more likely to experience spontaneous bleeding. Around 20 percent of women with severe FXI deficiency are at risk of experiencing severe bleeding after delivery if they do not receive treatment. Unlike other clotting factors, the level of FXI does not increase during pregnancy and may decrease in the third trimester and close to delivery [23–25].

Factor XIII (FXIII) is essential for stabilizing blood clots. Its subunit A facilitates the covalent bond between fibrin monomers, resulting in a stable clot that is protected from degradation. FXIII deficiency can be inherited or acquired. Severe congenital FXIII deficiency is rare, with a prevalence of 1 in 1–3 million live births. Individuals with congenital FXIII deficiency experience prolonged bleeding, as well as complications in wound healing, tissue repair, and extracellular matrix deposition.

Homozygotes or compound heterozygous subjects may exhibit prolonged bleeding from the umbilical stump, heavy menstrual bleeding, joint bleeding, intracranial hemorrhage, recurrent early pregnancy loss, and delayed postoperative and post-traumatic bleeding. Heterozygotes, on the other hand, are usually asymptomatic. Researchers have identified 153 mutations associated with FXIII deficiency, with missense variations occurring in about 50% of cases. In 95% of individuals with congenital FXIII deficiency, subunit A is undetectable, while subunit B is around 20–50%. The subunit B acts as a carrier of subunit A in circulation and protects it from spontaneous activation. Acquired FXIII deficiency is more prevalent and can be caused by various factors, including major surgeries, obstetric complications during delivery, ischemic stroke, acute myocardial infarction (MI), COVID-19 complications, trauma, autoimmune-mediated conditions such as lupus erythematosus and rheumatoid arthritis, and certain medications like valproic acid, tocilizumab, chemotherapeutic agents, and isoniazid. FXIII levels decrease continuously from the first trimester of pregnancy until delivery, although they remain within normal ranges. Some studies have found that FXIII levels are decreased in women experiencing blood loss greater than 500 mL compared to those with less blood loss, even when the factor levels are within normal ranges. Additionally, studies have shown that FXIII is the only factor influencing measured blood loss in postpartum hemorrhage (PPH) in previously asymptomatic women. Based on statistical models, increasing FXIII activity by 30% would result in a 39% reduction in PPH risk, and a 50% increase would decrease the risk of PPH by 73%. Although congenital FXIII deficiency is rare, researchers suggest including FXIII monitoring in standard measures to assess the risk of PPH [26]. A follow-up multicenter study in Switzerland aims to determine whether administration of FXIII concentrates in an early stage of PPH would reduce blood loss (NCT06481995).

Fibrinogen: The important role of fibrinogen in blood coagulation has been well documented. In non-pregnant women, the average fibrinogen level is 2–4 g/L, but during pregnancy, it increases to more than 5 g/L as an acute phase protein.

Several studies have shown that the fibrinogen level can decrease rapidly in cases of initial blood loss despite the increased coagulation typically observed during pregnancy. Cortet's prospective analysis highlighted the role of fibrinogen in the severity of postpartum hemorrhage (PPH). His study of 743 PPH cases demonstrated that fibrinogen levels were independently associated with PPH severity, with a significantly higher odds ratio for severe PPH (11.9; 2.56–56.06) for fibrinogen levels <2 g/L compared to 1.90 (1.16–3.09) for fibrinogen levels >2–3 [27].

Similar findings were reported by Charbit, whose analysis of 128 cases indicated that fibrinogen levels were the sole predictive factor for severe PPH. The positive predictive value of fibrinogen levels <2 g/L was 100%, while the negative predictive value of levels >4 g/L was 79% [28].

Hereditary fibrinogen disorders (HFD) include quantitative deficiencies such as hypofibrinogenemia and afibrinogenemia, as well as qualitative deficiencies like dysfibrinogenemia and hypodysfibrinogenemia. The prevalence of recessive fibrinogen deficiency is estimated to be 1–25 in 1,000,000, with prevalence influenced by ethnicity [29]. The clinical manifestations can range from asymptomatic to life-threatening bleeding, depending on the severity of the deficiency and some DNA variants. Although the level of fibrinogen increases during pregnancy, it does not reach the physiological levels characteristic of the end of pregnancy.

In a study by Hugon-Rodin, which analyzed 159 pregnancies with hypo-, dys-, and hypodysfibrinogenemia, postpartum hemorrhage (PPH) was observed in 62 pregnancies (19.9%). Obstetric complications were noticed in 17.3 percent of live births, including vaginal bleeding, retroplacental hematoma, and thrombosis [30]. Inherited afibrinogenemia occurs in 1 in 1,000,000, with bleeding symptoms usually present at birth. Individuals with this defect commonly experience bleeding symptoms like those of FXIII deficient patients, and in a minority, they may also be at risk of thrombosis. Women with inherited afibrinogenemia are at high risk of miscarriage, antepartum bleeding, and severe PPH [30].

The role of fibrinogen in coagulation is crucial, as it is the first coagulation factor to decrease in case of massive bleeding due to obstetric complications. Measuring fibrinogen levels close to delivery appears to be an effective predictor of primary PPH due to its significant role in coagulation. Inherited fibrinogen deficiency, except for afibrinogenemia, may be asymptomatic before pregnancy, leading to bleeding complications in 20–25% of pregnancies. This risk exists both with and without inherited fibrinogen deficiency. Due to the variability of risk factors influencing fast fibrinogen decrease during delivery and postpartum, both inherited and acquired fibrinogen deficiencies require equal attention. Rapid diagnosis of fibrinogen levels would increase the likelihood of directed factor replacement, particularly in the dynamic process of massive bleeding that may lead to fibrinogen deficiency caused by any inherited factor deficiency.

2.3 Timely diagnosis of coagulopathy in cases of postpartum hemorrhage (PPH) is crucial for effective management and positive patient outcomes

Owning the evidence of factors variability that could cause PPH, including symptoms that may potentially be overseen before pregnancy, screening questionnaires regarding emergency pregnancy and/or delivery would increase the attention to the inherent likelihood for primary and secondary PPH [31]. Rodeghiero et al. for the first time structured a bleeding questionnaire in the international multicenter study (IMS) to assess the impact of bleeding symptoms on the risk of developing PPH in women with a family history of autosomal dominant type I VWD and those without a bleeding disorder. The study showed 8 -fold higher risk for vaginal dilatation, blood transfusion, suturing, and a remarkably increased risk of undergoing a hysterectomy for PPH for women with VWD [32].

The ISTH bleeding assessment tool (BAT) was developed for screening individuals with bleeding symptoms to improve the diagnosis of VWD. In 2010, the International Society for Hemostasis and Thrombosis (ISTH) presented the BAT with a specificity of 75% and sensitivity of 54% available in English, German, Norwegian, Spanish, and Japanese. The specificity and sensitivity are the results of a systematic analysis of 7 studies that assessed the use of ISTH BAT for screening pediatrics and adults for VWD. The studies validated BAT by comparing the probability of VWD with laboratory tests for the diagnosis of VWD. The time necessary to answer the questions is 10 to 20, in some cases up to 30 minutes, depending on the experience of the operator. The ISTH BAT contains 14 questions on different types of bleeding symptoms with an assessment of intensity, length, and type of treatment needed. The score < 6 in adult females is normal and < 3 in children is normal [33].

The diagnosis of a possible bleeding disorder rests on the use of screening tests (aPTT, PT, fibrinogen, and platelet count) and second-level tests aimed at identifying the specific factor deficiency/abnormality. Historically, activated partial thromboplastin time (aPTT) is used to measure the time to generate fibrin from citrated plasma by adding an external agent, e.g., kaolin, to activate the intrinsic coagulation pathway. Prolonged aPTT can be caused by a deficiency of clotting factors involved in the intrinsic and common pathway (factors XII, XI, X, IX, VIII, V, prothrombin, and fibrinogen). Normal aPTT ranges from 21 to 35 seconds, but each laboratory should establish its own normal range. Similarly, the prothrombin time (PT) is used to assess the time to generate fibrin after activation of VII. Thromboplastin is added to citrated plasma to stimulate the extrinsic and common pathway in the 37°C incubation. Physiological PT is usually in the range of 12–15 seconds, but each laboratory should make its own normal range. Isolated PT prolongation is associated with FVII deficiency, while a combined prolongation of PT and aPTT is usually caused by the deficiency of FV, X, prothrombin, and fibrinogen. In addition, the citrated plasma can be stimulated by thrombin to trigger the transformation of fibrinogen to fibrin. This method is known as thrombin time (TT), whose prolongation points to a deficiency or abnormality of fibrinogen [34].

Besides the basic methods, measuring antigen and activity level is an important way to quantify coagulopathy. Enzyme-linked immunosorbent assays (ELISA) employing monoclonal antibodies are commonly used to measure the antigen concentration of VWF, while usually, for all other coagulopathies, activity measurement is easier and largely available. Levels of vWF: Ag and activity in type 1 vWD are similarly reduced, while in type 2 there is usually a discrepancy in the ratio of VWF activity/VWF:Ag (< 0.6) due to the presence of qualitative abnormality of the protein. In type 3, both VWF:Ag and activity are undetectable or very low (< 1–2 U/dL) [35].

Additional tests are used to detect the subtypes of vWD due to the variation of vWD mutations. Ristocetin cofactor (RCo) assay and ristocetin-induced platelet agglutination (RIPA) are qualitative methods to distinguish Type 2 VWD. Enhanced RIPA, which occurs at concentrations lower than in normal controls, is characteristic of Type 2B VWD. Genetic testing could confirm the diagnostic based on the abovementioned test and additionally support the family diagnostic.

FXIII deficiency is not detectable using the usual screening tests (aPTT, PT), and a specific assay is required in the presence of a clinical suspicion. Specialized tests include FXIII activity and antigen assay, clot solubility test, and genetic test [36].

Thromboelastography (TEG) and rotational rhromboelastometry (ROTEM) are viscoelastic methods providing numerical and graphical presentation of induced hemostasis from whole blood. Several studies showed an effective and timely diagnosis of fibrinogen deficiency by using ROTEM in obstetrics, resulting in reduced blood loss [37]. The implementation of viscoelastic tests in obstetrics could increase the likelihood of effective management of PPH considering the variation of measures, including coagulation factor activation, factor amplification and fibrin cross-linking, clot strength, maximal clot strength, and fibrinolysis, which offers the ability to manage fibrinogen deficiency, FXIII deficiency, and possibly platelet dysfunction [37, 38].

Moreover, new technologies in development could possibly assist in monitoring coagulation factor levels quickly and accurately. A group of researchers from the medical university in Ankara and NANODEV Scientific are currently validating a portable device for measuring the level of fibrinogen from whole blood using surface plasmon resonance (SRPR) technology. This could potentially be used for measuring any protein and might be feasible for high and low-resource settings [39].

2.4 Treatment options and protocols

Considering the changes of coagulation factors that occur during pregnancy in women with inherited bleeding disorders, the variations in their phenotype and genotype, using the BAT or another screening questionnaire for bleeding symptoms at the beginning of pregnancy could potentially help identify women who require close

	week 35	delivery	1-week postpartum	8 weeks postpartum	>12 weeks postpartum
VWF % of normal	262(95–718)	376(133–1064)	351	93	78
FVIII % of normal*	no data published	no data published	no data published	no data published	67
FIX% of normal*	no data published	no data published	no data published	no data published	65
FXI% of normal	71(±11)	56(±14)	no data available	76(±11)	96(± 5)
FXIII% of normal	83(±21)**	no data published	90(±19)***	no data published	no data published
	levels at week 35	delivery	5 weeks postpartum		normal
Fibrinogen g/L	5.4 ± 0.8	5.7 ± 0.7	3.1 ± 0.7		2.4-4.2

**Carriers of hemophilia.*
***Levels in the third trimester.*
****Levels postpartum.*

Table 1.
Summary of factor values in pregnancy and post-partum [40, 41].

monitoring of essential coagulation factors for the prevention of postpartum hemorrhage (PPH) (**Table 1**). Women with von Willebrand disease (VWD) should undergo monitoring at least in the third trimester for VWF: RCo and FVIII:C levels. It would be preferable if genetic testing could support the direct treatment, especially in cases of DNA variants with increased clearance of VWF that prevent the achievement of normal levels by the end of pregnancy. Considering the limited availability of genetic testing, the availability of desmopressin test results before pregnancy would help in deciding the appropriate preventive treatment before and after delivery. In general, women with VWD type 1 who achieve FVIII: C or VWF levels lower than 50 IU/dL in the third trimester should receive desmopressin immediately after delivery and for the following 3–4 days. Type 2A and type 2B VWD typically require replacement of VWF with VWF/FVIII concentrate or with recombinant VWF, which has recently been approved by EMA, FDA, and Swissmedic. In Type 2 B with platelet count <30–50,000/uL at time of parturition, platelet concentrate administration should also be considered. Similarly, VWD type 2 M and type 3 should be treated with VWF concentrates. VWD type 2 N can be safely managed with desmopressin.

Individuals with FVIII and FIX deficiency should be monitored during pregnancy, and their factor levels should be checked at weeks 23 and 34, as well as before any invasive procedures. Depending on their factor levels, they should be treated with FVIII and FIX concentrates or a desmopressin dose of 0.3 μg/pregnancy weight before delivery.

Historically, the threshold for prophylactic factor correction has been an activity level of 50 IU/dL, although a study by Punt et al. found no difference in the occurrence of PPH in those who received prophylactic treatment compared to those who did not [19]. According to WFH guidelines, concentrates of FVIII and IX are recommended, with the target level for FVIII being 1.0 IU/mL and not falling below 0.5 IU/mL. Factor IX level correction is also recommended using factor concentrates. For the insertion and removal of an epidural catheter for spinal anesthesia, both FVIII and IX levels should be above 0.5 IU/mL. In cases where FVIII or FIX is less than 0.5 IU/mL, it is recommended to administer tranexamic acid of 1000 mg before delivery [42].

FXIII levels decrease during pregnancy, and some studies have shown the impact of prepartum FXIII levels on blood loss, with an increase of each unit of FXIII activity level linked to maintaining blood loss below 500 mL. However, FXIII is usually not checked in normal women before delivery. Severe forms of FXIII deficiency should receive prophylactic replacement therapy during pregnancy. FXIII is available as a plasma-derived concentrate or recombinant, with the recommended dose being 15–20 IU/kg [43].

The historical data on the impact of FXI deficiency on the occurrence of PPH is unbalanced. While FXI deficiency did not trigger PPH in vaginal delivery, women with a mild form of FXI deficiency who underwent cesarean section were found to have a twofold higher likelihood of experiencing PPH compared to the controls [44]. FXI deficiency is recommended to be managed by antifibrinolytics (such as tranexamic acid), fresh frozen plasma, FXI concentrates, and rFVIIa. There have been documented cases in the literature of thromboembolic complications following the use of plasma-derived FXI concentrates. In the early 90s, an antithrombin agent was added to the manufacturing process to minimize the risk of complications. Generally, the use of FXI concentrates should be carefully considered in women with thromboembolic risk. Moreover, for individuals with an increased risk or with inhibitors against FXI, rFVIIa could be used for the management of PPH [45, 46].

Fibrinogen deficiency has gained attention in the last decade in the context of acute bleeding. Inherited deficiencies/abnormalities can cause postpartum hemorrhage (PPH), especially if not recognized or treated. In addition, special attention should be given to any massive bleeding, as even mild forms of acquired hypofibrinogenemia (fibrinogen level < 200 mg/dL) during delivery can cause significant blood loss.

The introduction of TEG and ROTEM has significantly improved the diagnosis of acquired fibrinogen deficiency in cardiac surgery, trauma, and obstetrics settings. Despite the lack of clear consensus for optimal fibrinogen levels during pregnancy and delivery, historically published data suggests that the fibrinogen level should be maintained at ≥0.5–0.6 g/L during pregnancy and ≥ 1.0–1.5 g/L during delivery [47]. Fibrinogen is available as a plasma-derived concentrate with presentations of 1 G or 2 G per vial.

A small group of institutions recently published their protocols for the treatment of massive bleeding during and postpartum. Examples of implementing patients' blood management in PPH as a concept of a multidisciplinary approach have shown positive outcomes. For instance, Luzern Kanton Hospital in Switzerland has been following the PPH management protocol since 2015 with updates in 2020 and 2024.

This protocol recommends point-of-care measurement of missing coagulation factors (ROTEM) if the blood loss is <1000 mL. Specific treatment is recommended for blood loss >1000 mL. A fibrinogen level < 2 g/L during delivery is perceived as a risk factor for developing PPH. The advocated dose of fibrinogen concentrate (FC) is 30–60 mg/kg (2–4-8 g) with the aim of achieving a fibrinogen level of 2 g/L. FC can be administered in parallel or as an alternative to fresh frozen plasma (FFP) at a dose of 20–30 ml/kg. If not effective, the recommended treatment step includes the administration of 25 IU/kg body weight of prothrombin complex concentrate, which consists of factors II, VII, X, and IX. Desmopressin is advised to be administered at a dosage of 0.3 μg/kg body weight every 12–24 hours, but not longer than a couple of days due to the risk of hyponatremia and tachyphylaxis with loss of response [48].

Similarly, the Santa Joana group of Hospitals in Sao Paulo, Brazil, introduced their protocol for PPH in 2013. According to the protocol, they measure the fibrinogen level upon admission. If it is less than 2 g/L or 1.5 g/L, they administer 2 or 4 g of FC, respectively. The institution also includes measurements of hemoglobin and platelet count as potential predictive factors for the risk of PPH [49].

2.5 Guidelines for PPH management

The complexity of inherited coagulopathies increases the risk of developing PPH if they are not already diagnosed and properly managed. Significant reduction in some coagulation factors can lead to acute massive blood loss, prompting experts to recommend management algorithms for PPH. In 2023, Hoffer and colleagues suggested close monitoring of coagulation factors using viscoelastic tests like TEG or ROTEM when blood loss is ≥500 mL. They recommended administering 1 g of tranexamic acid if blood loss exceeds 1000 mL within 3 hours. Additionally, they proposed an initial dose of 4 g of fibrinogen concentrate if levels are ≤2 g/l or FIBTEM 5A ≤ 12 mm. A massive transfusion protocol (MTP) is suggested for blood loss >2500 mL [50].

In 2006, the UK Hemophilia Center's Doctor Organization recommended a multidisciplinary team of hematologists, obstetricians, and anesthesiologists for managing pregnancy in carriers of hemophilia, aligning with the above information [51].

The Australian consensus statement advises monitoring coagulation factors during pregnancy, particularly at weeks 32–34, and correcting coagulopathy to prevent PPH. They also recommend administering 1 g of tranexamic acid before delivery and paying attention to the epidural catheter and intramuscular application when coagulation factor levels are <50 IU/dL [52].

Various gynecology and obstetrics associations under FIGO suggest managing the uterine tonus as the primary cause of PPH. Fibrinogen replacement is recommended when levels are below 2 g/L, aiming to achieve levels of 1.5–2.0 g/L [53].

The diversity of recommendations for PPH management underscores the importance of a multidisciplinary approach. However, achieving a common consensus and implementing these recommendations may be challenging, especially in low- and middle-income countries. Therefore, the WHO released its first road map to combat PPH in 2023, with plans to publish consolidated guidelines in 2025.

2.6 New treatment options in inherited bleeding disorders: What applies to PPH?

The quality of life for individuals with hemophilia has notably improved over the last two decades due to the development of extended half-life products, non-factor replacement therapies, and recently approved gene therapy. However, challenges in treating inherited bleeding disorders remain a burden for patients, caregivers, and healthcare systems, particularly in low- and middle-income countries.

Emicizumab is a humanized bispecific monoclonal antibody that binds together FIXa and FX, mimicking the function of missing activated FVIII in individuals with FVIII deficiency. Emicizumab is approved by the U.S. Food and Drug Administration (FDA), European Medicines Agency (EMA), and Swiss medicine and is registered in many countries in the USA, Europe, Latin America, Turkey, and the Middle East. It is indicated for the prophylactic treatment of hemophilia A in individuals with or without inhibitors against FVIII. A clinical trial is currently underway to investigate the use of emicizumab in the treatment of VWD type 3 (NCT 05500807). Currently, there is no available data on the use of emicizumab in pregnancy and as a prophylactic treatment for PPH [54, 55].

Concizumab and marstacimab are monoclonal antibodies, administered subcutaneously, that target tissue factor pathway inhibitor to enhance thrombin generation. Clinical trials have demonstrated their efficacy and safety in patients with hemophilia A and B, with and without inhibitors. Concizumab has recently been approved by the Canadian health authority, Swissmedic, EMA, and in Japan. Similarly, marstacimab is approved by the FDA and EMA. However, data on the use of these agents in pregnancy and for the prevention and treatment of PPH is not available.

Fitusiran, a small interfering RNA, acts on antithrombin (AT) mRNA in the liver to block AT translation. When administered monthly as a subcutaneous injection, it improves thrombin generation and leads to a reduction in bleeding episodes in individuals with hemophilia A and B. However, its use in pregnancy and for the prevention and treatment of PPH has not been investigated.

Serpin PC is an investigational recombinant serine protease inhibitor developed specifically to inhibit activated protein C (APC). Currently, there is a Phase II study ongoing in 55 centers aiming to enroll 120 individuals with severe and moderately severe hemophilia, with or without inhibitors (NCT05798524). The population of interest in this chapter, however, is not included in the clinical trial.

Gene therapies for the treatment of hemophilia A and B have been developed with the aim of overcoming the challenges in managing these inherited conditions, potentially allowing patients to move to a mild form or non-hemophilic status. In this approach, the capsid of the adeno-associated virus is used as a carrier of the transgene, directed to the liver to produce the missing FVIII or FIX in hepatocytes. Gene therapy for hemophilia A and B involves a single intravenous administration. The therapy for hemophilia B is currently approved in the USA, Canada, EMA, and has been recommended for use by the National Institute for Health and Care Excellence (NICE) in the UK, Swiss Medic, and Japan. Similarly, the gene therapy for hemophilia A has been approved by the FDA and EMA. Both therapies are currently being investigated for the treatment of hemophilia A and B in adult males with severe deficiency, with no data available on their use in women.

In addition to viral capsid vector-based gene replacement technology, there are other alternatives for hemophilia and VWD in development. These include clustered regularly interspaced short palindromic repeats (CRISPR)/Cas9 gene editing technology in VWD Type 2 N and hemophilia B, using an adeno-associated viral vector (AAV). Another technology being explored is the use of lipid nanoparticles and small interfering RNA (siRNA) delivery systems for further development in the treatment of hemophilia A and B [56, 57].

3. Conclusion

Notable efforts have been made to reduce maternal mortality by introducing the WHO road map, new bleeding management approaches, and diagnostic and treatment options. However, significant challenges still exist, especially in low-resource settings. A multidisciplinary approach involving hematologists, obstetricians, and anesthesiologists in each case of massive blood loss during delivery, regardless of a history of inherited bleeding disorders, should be established. Women with inherited bleeding disorders should be managed accordingly, and plans for managing delivery should be established before/at the beginning of pregnancy. Ideally, a treatment protocol for managing PPH should support institutions and assistants (such as midwives and health helpers) to prevent life-threatening blood loss. New diagnostic tools currently in development hold promise for timely diagnosis and targeted treatment for women experiencing blood loss during and after delivery. It is likely that the population at risk of PPH, regardless of a history of bleeding disorders, will not be included in clinical trials for new treatments in development, so it may not significantly change the current treatment options. Furthermore, gaining real-world experience in using recently approved treatments for PPH would help enhance recommendations and improve clinical outcomes for women at risk of PPH.

Acknowledgements

I would like to thank M. Punt and R. Wyss for their input and comments on this work. The open access was supported by CSL Behring.

Conflict of interest

No conflict of interest. Jolana Schmiedl is the employee of CSL Behring.

Author details

Jolana Schmiedl[1*] and Giancarlo Castaman[2]

1 CSL Behring, Bern, Switzerland

2 Center for Bleeding Disorders and Coagulation, Department of Oncology, Careggi University Hospital, Florence, Italy

*Address all correspondence to: jolanaschmiedl@gmail.com

References

[1] World Health Organisation. [Internet]. 26 Apr 2024. Available from: https://www.who.int/news-room/fact-sheets/detail/maternal-mortality [Accessed: November 26, 2024]

[2] World Health Organisation. Trends in Maternal Mortality 2000 to 2020: Estimates by WHO, UNICEF, UNFPA, World Bank Group and UNDESA/Population Division [Internet]. 23 Feb 2023. Available from: https://www.who.int/data/gho/indicator-metadata-registry/imr-details/9789240068759 [Accessed: November 26, 2024]

[3] Hoyert DL. Maternal Mortality Rates in the United States. National Center of Health Statistics; 2022. Available from: https://www.cdc.gov/nchs/data/hestat/maternal-mortality/2022/maternal-mortality-rates-2022.pdf

[4] van der Akker T et al. Prioritizing actions to address maternal mortality rates globally. Lancet. 3 Feb 2024;**403**(10425):417-419. DOI: 10.1016/S0140-6736(23)02290-0. Epub 2023 Oct 27

[5] Yang Y et al. Factors associated with primary post-partum hemorrhage in elderly women undergoing repeated cesarean delivery. International Journal of Women's Health. 29 Dec 2021;**13**:1261-1267. DOI: 10.2147/IJWH.S332020

[6] WHO. A roadmap to combat postpartum hemorrhage between 2023 and 2030. 2023. Available from: https://www.who.int/publications/i/item/9789240081802

[7] Schmiedl J, Castaman G. Awareness of von Willebrand disease among gynecologists: Investigating the referral of women with heavy menstrual bleeding to hematologists. IJGO. 2024;**167**:453-455. DOI: 10.1002/ijgo.15546

[8] Lavin M. Significant gynecological bleeding in women with low von Willebrand factor levels. Blood Advances. 24 Jul 2018;**2**(14):1784-1791

[9] Bestman PL. A comparative analysis of postpartum hemorrhage incidence and influencing factors between nulliparous and multiparous women in Hunan Province, China: A multicenter retrospective cohort study. Preventive Medicine Reports. 10 Jan 2024;**38**:102580. DOI: 10.1016/j.pmedr.2023.102580. eCollection 2024 Feb

[10] Zhang WC. Meta-analysis to assess the role of maternal characteristics and risk factors on postpartum hemorrhage. Advances in Clinical and Experimental Medicine. Jul 2023;**32**(7):723-731. DOI: 10.17219/acem/158474

[11] Wormer KC et al. Acute Post Partum Hemorrhage. National Library of Medicine; 2023. PMID: 29763164. Bookshelf ID: NBK499988. Available from: https://pubmed.ncbi.nlm.nih.gov/29763164/

[12] Agiq F et al. Major differences in clinical presentation, diagnosis and management of men and women with autosomal inherited bleeding disorders. EClinicalMedicine. 29 Jan 2021;**32**:100726. DOI: 10.1016/j.eclinm.2021.100726. eCollection 2021 Feb

[13] Kirtava A et al. Medical, reproductive, and psychosocial experiences of women diagnosed with von Willebrand's disease receiving care in hemophilia treatment centers: A case-control study. Haemophilia. Jun 2003;**9**(3):292-297

[14] Sladic M, Verdenik I, Smrkolj S. The effect on von Willebrand pregnancy, delivery, and post-partum period: A retrospective observational study. Medicina. 2022;**58**(6):774. DOI: 10.3390/medicina58060774

[15] Castaman G. Changes of von Willebrand factor during pregnancy in women with and without von Willebrand disease. Mediterranean Journal of Hematology and Infectious Diseases. 16 Jul 2013;**5**(1):e2013052. DOI: 10.4084/MJHID.2013.052

[16] Castaman G et al. Pregnancy and delivery in women with von Willebrand disease and different von Willebrand factor mutations. Haematologica. 30 Nov 2009;**95**(6):963-969. DOI: 10.3324/haematol.2009.011239

[17] Castaman G et al. Pregnancy and delivery in patients with heterozygous and homozygous R8456Q type 2N von Willebrand disease. Journal of Thrombosis and Haemostasis. Feb 2005;**3**(2):391-392. DOI: 10.1111/j.1538-7836.2005.01162.x

[18] Lack M et al. Clinical manifestations and complications of childbirth and replacement therapy in 385 Iranian patients with type 3 von Willebrand disease. British Journal of Haematology. 2000;**111**(4):1236-1239

[19] Punt M. Maternal and neonatal bleeding complications in relation to peripartum management in hemophilia carriers: A systematic review. Blood Reviews Journal. 2024. Article in press. Available from: www.elsevier.com/locate/issn/0268960X

[20] Plug I. Bleeding in carriers of hemophilia. Blood. 1 Jul 2006;**108**(1):52-56. DOI: 10.1182/blood-2005-09-3879

[21] Stoof SCM et al. Primary postpartum hemorrhage in women with von Willebrand disease or carriership of hemophilia despite care: A retrospective survey. Haemophilia. Jul 2015;**21**(4):505-512. DOI: 10.1111/hae.12635

[22] Mohammed MB et al. An update on FXI structure and function. DOI: 10.1016/j.thromres.2017.10.008

[23] Zhang X et al. Global epidemiology of factor XI deficiency: A targeted review of the literature and foundation reports. DOI: 10.1111/hae.14687

[24] Asselta R et al. Exploring the global landscape of genetic variation in coagulation factor XI deficiency. Blood. 27 Jul 2017;**130**(4):e1-e6. DOI: 10.1182/blood-2017-04-780148

[25] Wheeler AP et al. The clinical management of factor XI deficiency in pregnant women. Expert Review of Hematology. Jul 2020;**13**(7):719-729. DOI: 10.1080/17474086.2020.1772745

[26] Haslinger C et al. The impact of pre partum FXIII activity on post-partum blood los. Journal of Thrombosis and Haemostasis. Jun 2020;**18**(6):1310-1319. DOI: 10.1111/jth.14795

[27] Cortet M et al. Association between fibrinogen level and severity of postpartum hemorrhage: Secondary analysis of a prospective trial. British Journal of Anaesthesia. 2012;**108**(6):984-989. DOI: 10.1093/bja/aes096

[28] Charbit B et al. The decrease of fibrinogen is an early predictor of the severity of postpartum hemorrhage. Journal of Thrombosis and Haemostasias. 2007;**5**:266-273

[29] Ramanan R. Congenital fibrinogen disorders: Strengthening genotype–phenotype correlations through novel genetic diagnostic tools. British Journal of Haematology. 2023;**203**(3):355-368. DOI: 10.1111/bjh.19039

[30] Hugon-Rodin J. Obstetrical complications in hereditary fibrinogen disorders: The Fibrinogest study. Journal of Thrombosis and Haemostasis. Aug 2023;**21**(8):2126-2136. DOI: 10.1016/j.jtha.2023.04.035

[31] Siboni SM, Spreafico M, Calo L, et al. Gynecological and obstetrical problems in women with different bleeding disorders. Haemophilia. 2009;**15**:1291-1299. Available from: https://radiologykey.com/postpartum-hemorrhage/

[32] Rodeghiero F, Castaman G, Tosetto A, Batlle J, Baudo F, Cappelletti A, et al. The discriminant power of bleeding history for the diagnosis of type 1 von Willebrand disease: An international, multicenter study. Journal of Thrombosis and Haemostasis. 2005;**3**:2619-2626. DOI: 10.1111/j.1538-7836.2005.01663.x

[33] Kalot MA et al. Bleeding assessment tool in the diagnosis of VWD in adults and children: Systematic review and meta-analysis of accuracy. Blood Advances. 2021;**5**(23):5023-5031

[34] Raber MN. Coagulation tests. In: Walker HK, Hall WD, Hurst JW, editors. Clinical Methods: The History, Physical, and Laboratory Examinations. Chapter 157. 3rd ed. Boston: Butterworths; 1990. Available from: https://www.ncbi.nlm.nih.gov/books/NBK265/

[35] Furlong RA et al. The combined use of monoclonal antibody-based enzyme-linked immunosorbent assays (ELISA) for factor VIII antigen (VIII:Ag) and von Willebrand factor antigen (vWF:Ag) for the detection of carriers of hemophilia a. Clinical & Laboratory Haematology. 1988;**10**(3):295-305. DOI: 10.1111/j.1365-2257.1988.tb00023.x

[36] Mangla A et al. Factor XIII deficiency. National Library of Medicine. In: StatPearls [Internet]. Treasure Island, FL: StatPearls Publishing; Jan 2024. Available from: https://www.ncbi.nlm.nih.gov/books/NBK557467/

[37] Amgalan A. Systematic review of viscoelastic testing (TEG/ROTEM) in obstetrics and recommendations from the women's SSC of the ISTH. Journal of Thrombosis and Haemostasis. Aug 2020;**18**(8):1813-1838. DOI: 10.1111/jth.14882

[38] Mascio N. Thromboelastometry – Guided treatment algorithm in post- partum hemorrhage. British Journal of Anaesthesia. 14 Mar 2023;**130**(6):e456-e458. DOI: 10.1016/j.bja.2023.02.012

[39] Cimen D. Real-time detection of fibrinogen via imprinted recognition sites. ChemistrySelect. 2021;**6**(35):9435-9441. DOI: 10.1002/slct.202101942

[40] Bremme KA. Hemostatic changes in pregnancy. Best Practice & Research Clinical Haematology. Jun 2003;**16**(2):153-168. DOI: 10.1016/S1521-6926(03)00021-5

[41] Sharief LT. Changes in factor XIII level during pregnancy. Haemophilia. Mar 2014;**20**(2):e144-8. DOI: 10.1111/hae.12345. Epub 2013 Dec 16. PMID: 24329777

[42] Rodriguez MF. Carriers of hemophilia: Pregnancy, childbirth, and post-partum. Blood Coagul Fibrinolysis. 1 Dec 2020;**31**(1S):S9-S11. DOI: 10.1097/MBC.0000000000000989

[43] Duque P, Korte W. FXIII in the acute care setting and its relevance in obstetric bleeding. Transfusion Medicine and Hemotherapy. 24 Nov 2022;**50**(1):10-17. DOI: 10.1159/000526489

[44] Bogue T et al. Pops-partum hemorrhage outcomes in women with mold FXI deficiency. Blood. Nov 2019;**134**(Suppl. 1):629-629. DOI: 10.1182/blood-2019-124759

[45] Maggs B. Factor XI deficiency and its management. Hemophilia. 2000;**6**(Supplement. 1):100-1009

[46] Bern MM et al. Treatment of factor XI inhibitors using recombinant activated FVIa. Haemophilia. Jan 2005;**11**(1):20-25. DOI: 10.1111/j.1365-2516.2005.01052.x

[47] Saes JL. Pregnancy outcome in afibrinogenemia: Are we giving enough fibrinogen concentrate? A case series. Research and Practice in Thrombosis and Haemostasis. 22 Jan 2020;**4**(2):343-346 DOI: 10.1002/rth2.12300

[48] Krischer B, Uerlings V. Luzerner Kantonalspital. 2024. Available from: https://www.obsgyn-wiki.ch/geburtszentrum/fachliche-weisungen/postpartale-haemorrhagie

[49] Siaulys MM. Manual de Anestesia obstétricia. Grupo Santa Joana. 2024. pp. 78-99. Available from: https://www.evoluthe.com.br/p-19006931-Manual-De-Anestesia-Obstetrica---Monica-M.-Siaulys. ISBN 9788520458730

[50] Hoffer S et al. Hemostatic support in postpartum hemorrhage a review of the literature and expert opinion. European Journal of Anaesthesiology. 1 Jan 2023;**40**(1):29-38. DOI: 10.1097/EJA.0000000000001744

[51] Lee CA. The obstetric and gynaecological management of women with inherited bleeding disorders – review with guidelines produced by a taskforce of UK Haemophilia Centre Doctors Organization. Haemophilia. 2006;**12**:301-336. DOI: 10.1111/j.1365-2516.2006.01314.x

[52] Dunkley S et al. Updated Australian consensus statement on management of inherited bleeding disorders in pregnancy. The Medical Journal of Australia. Apr 2019;**210**(7):326-332. DOI: 10.5694/mja2.50123

[53] Escobar MF. FIGO recommendations on the management of post- partum hemorrhage. IJGO. 2022;**157**(S1):3-50. DOI: 10.1002/ijgo.14116

[54] Parisi K, Kumar A. Emicizumab. Available from: https://www.ncbi.nlm.nih.gov/books/NBK559180/

[55] Kruse-Jarres RT et al. Surgical outcomes in people with hemophilia a taking emicizumab prophylaxis: Experience from the HAVE 1-4 study. Blood Advances. 27 Dec 2022;**6**(24):6140-6150. DOI: 10.1182/bloodadvances.2022007458

[56] Shi Q et al. A novel mouse model in type 2N VWD was developed by CRISPR/Cas9 gene editing and recapitulates human type 2N VWD. Blood Advances. 10 May 2022;**6**(9):2778-2790. DOI: 10.1182/bloodadvances.2021006353

[57] Chernyi N et al. Recent advances in gene therapy for hemophilia: Projecting the perspective. Biomolecules. 2024;**14**(7):854. DOI: 10.3390/biom14070854